The Essential Yoga Sutra

by the same authors

*The Diamond Cutter: The Buddha on Strategies
for Managing Your Business and Your Life**

*The Tibetan Book of Yoga**

*The Garden: A Parable**

How Yoga Works

The 18 Books of the Foundation Series
Asian Classics Institute

The 10 Meditation Modules
Asian Classics Institute

*published by Doubleday

Three Leaves Press

Doubleday   New York

The Essential
Yoga Sutra

*Ancient Wisdom
for Your Yoga*

Geshe Michael Roach and
Christie McNally

PUBLISHED BY DOUBLEDAY
a division of Random House, Inc.

Doubleday is a registered trademark and
Three Leaves Press and colophon are
trademarks of Random House, Inc.

Book design by Jennifer Ann Daddio

Library of Congress Cataloging-in-Publication Data

Roach, Michael, 1952–
    The essential Yoga sutra : ancient wisdom for your yoga /
Geshe Michael Roach and Christie McNally.—1st Three Leaves Press ed.
        p. cm.
    In English and Sanskrit (romanized); includes translation from
Sanskrit.
    Includes index.
    (alk. paper)
    1. Pataäjali. Yogasåtra. 2. Yoga—Early works to 1800. I. McNally,
Christie. II. Patañjali. Yogasutra. English & Sanskrit. III. Title.
B132. Y6P24337 2005   2004062090

ISBN 0-385-51536-7

PRINTED IN THE UNITED STATES OF AMERICA

July 2005
First Three Leaves Press Edition

10 9 8

Dedicated to the memory of

Samuel D. Atkins

(1911–2002)

Professor of Sanskrit;

Chairman, Department of Classics,

Princeton University;

and a good man

Contents

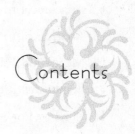

Second Cornerstone:
The Chapter on the Way

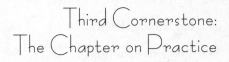

Third Cornerstone:
The Chapter on Practice

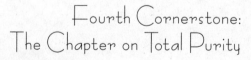

Fourth Cornerstone:
The Chapter on Total Purity

Foreword

We encourage readers to study the "Index of Important Ideas" at the end of this book, so that you know immediately where to look for help on any personal needs or interests you may have.

To help those who might want to chant the Yoga Sutra in its original language, we have included the Sanskrit here in the closest English pronunciation possible without special marks or spellings not found in normal English. Please note that the combination *a-a* should be read as one long *ah* sound. Divisions like this are made wherever two words are joined, but only if it would not change the pronunciation or meter in chanting.

The authors would like to acknowledge the kind assistance of the Asian Classics Input Project and its director, John Brady, for access to its database of several thousand ancient Asian manuscripts for completing this translation of the Yoga Sutra.

We would also like to thank Dr. M. A. Jayashree and Dr. M. A. Narasimhan, of the University of Mysore and University of Bangalore, India, for sharing with us their research on alternate readings from early handwritten and palm-leaf manuscripts of the Yoga Sutra. Ven. Brian K. Smith, PhD, a professor who teaches these materials at the University of California, Riverside; Loyola Marymount University; and Diamond Mountain University, carefully collated for us the variations of the Sanskrit text.

Finally, we would like to express infinite thanks to our many teachers from India, Tibet, and the West, who have spent thousands of hours patiently passing these teachings on to us.

Yogi, Dancer, Thinker, Doctor

A Short Book about Yoga:
The Yoga Sutra of Master Patanjali

Patanjala Yoga Sutram

A sutra is a short book that tells us the very crux of something—ideas tied tight together, with a stitch of thread. The Yoga Sutra is the mother book of all yoga. It was written about two thousand years ago by Master Patanjali.

Master Patanjali was a great yogi; he knew the physical poses of yoga and the art of breathing: yoga of the body. He was also a great thinker and meditator—a master of the yoga of the mind. He wrote as well famous books on medicine and on Sanskrit, the ancient tongue from which almost all our languages come. He is recognized too as the father of the classical dance of India.

Dancer, doctor, yogi, thinker, master of ancient words. What do they all have in common?

Yoga, as we shall see, has many meanings. One is the union of the winds within our inner body. We unite these winds with our yoga, when we think and understand. The winds will sing within us, the very first words of all. They will flow free, and force us to dance, and to run to heal others.

First Cornerstone

The Chapter on Meditation

2 It Begins with Meditation

Prathamah Samadhi Padah

The Yoga Sutra has four chapters: four cornerstones upon which it stands, like a table on four legs.

The first chapter describes five crucial steps that we all pass through during our spiritual journey. This journey always begins from pain: we see death, we see people suffer, we dream of saving them. And the journey ends when we change, finally, into a sacred being who actually has the power to save them.

In between its beginning and its end, the road we travel has five parts: five paths, each one leading into the next, each one marked by its own special milestones. Stepping up to each new path from the one before it can only be done in one way. We must be in deep meditation; we must learn to meditate.

Thus it is that the first chapter, the chapter on the five paths, is called the Chapter on Meditation.

3 The Power of Humility

I.1 I will now review for you
how we become whole.

Atha yoga-anushashanam.

Another meaning of yoga is to become whole. Ultimately we only become whole when we are truly capable of helping others with the things that really matter: when we can help them understand how they came into this world, and what life is for, and whether it has to end with losing everything.

This then, says Master Patanjali, is why I write my short book. He wants us to know, from the very beginning, that his book contains something of ultimate importance, something worth the precious hours of our life.

And I will only *review*, says the Master, what I have heard from my holy teachers. He attacks his own pride: I have nothing new to tell you, and there is nothing here that I have made up myself. I am only a vessel for the wisdom of the ages, and I pass it on to you—tried, tested, and unadulterated.

And he says "I will" write this book, for once a Master promises to do something, he does it—or dies trying.

All the great books of India begin with these three noble themes. Their power, their karma, stops all obstacles to the work we now begin.

4 To Become Whole

I.2 We become whole by stopping how the mind turns.

Yogash chitta virtti nirodhah.

These are perhaps the most important words of the entire Yoga Sutra. Here the Master tells us another meaning of yoga, which is learning to stop the Great Mistake.

And what is the Great Mistake? Our mind turns; meaning it turns things around the wrong way. A mother takes her small child to a movie. On the screen, a man is hurting a puppy.

The child cries out, and reaches to stop the man. Perhaps the child can even get up to the screen, and try to hit the man.

But this doesn't stop the man; it has nothing to do with the man. And the child hurts her own hand in the process.

Our mind makes this same kind of mistake, every day, every moment of every day. We need to stop the mistake, and that is yoga. Pain is real—yes—and it really hurts people. But we can only stop it if we can stop misunderstanding where it comes from. And this is what the Yoga Sutra teaches us to do.

5 The Seer

*I.3-4 On that day
the seer comes to dwell
within his own real nature.
Otherwise it follows
the form of the turning.*

*Tada drashtuh svarupevasthanam.
Virtti sarupyam itaratra.*

The most important day in our spiritual journey is the day that we first stop the Great Mistake. We stop seeing things the wrong way. The child realizes that the bad man is not really on the movie screen.

It only lasts for a brief time, the first time. And then, despite ourselves, we go back to making the same old mental mistake. But for a few minutes, we see the way we really are: we see that we are not at all the way we always thought we were.

These precious minutes, our first contact with the ultimate reality, are thus called the Path of Seeing. Not because we see these things with our eyes, but because we see them in very deep meditation, with our mind.

Until the day we see, our life continues to follow after the tragic mistake our mind is making, turning things around the wrong way. Until the child sees how things really are, she strikes out at the bad man on the screen, hurting herself and her mother too.

6 A Day in the Mind

*I.5–6 The mind turns
in five different ways.
They can be involved with afflictions
or free of them.
The five are correct perceptions,
mistaken perceptions, imagination, sleep, and memories.*

*Virttayah panchatayyah klishta-aklishtah.
Pramana viparyaya vikalpa nidra smirtayah.*

In a general sense, the mind turns or operates in many different ways: the ancient books of India list hundreds of different mental functions. Here though the Master chooses to deal with only five states of mind because, in a typical twenty-four-hour day, our mind will always be in one of these five states.

That is, we are usually seeing most things correctly, throughout the day. (It's true that I may misunderstand *how* I am, but not *that* I am.) Occasionally though we do make mistakes about what we see, and we bang the car.

We use our imagination to plan or to daydream, and we spend a good part of each day in sleep. We constantly call on our memories.

Our states of mind are sometimes stained by negative thoughts, thoughts that afflict us and make us unhappy. The ultimate negative thought is that same Great Mistake.

The goal of our yoga is not to stop all thoughts—that would be like throwing the baby out with the bathwater. We simply want to stop the mistake, and all the unhappiness it causes. We want to make our minds ultimately clear, and happy, and loving.

7 Right Seeing

*I.7 The different types of correct perception
are those that are direct,
deductive, or based on authority.*

Pratyaksha-anumana-agamah pramanani.

The vast majority of all that we see we see correctly. Even in the first few minutes out of bed in the morning, we have already had hundreds of correct perceptions: the sun is shining, these are my socks, breakfast smells good.

Correct perceptions are strong. Once we see something with a correct perception, we can truly say that thing exists.

These correct perceptions come in three types. Most of them are the direct type. I see a color, I hear a sound, I smell or taste or touch something. Hearing our thoughts in our own minds is also a direct type of correct perception.

Deduction is another kind of correct perception: I may not be able to see my socks on the floor in the morning, if they're covered by my pants. But if I dropped them there last night and I've had no visitors in the meantime, I know the socks are there, as surely as if I see them.

The last kind of correct perception is based on authority: I'm in my bedroom and can't see the kitchen, but Mother tells me there's still some breakfast left. And I know it's there, because she's a truthful person.

8 A Leaf in the Road

*I.8 Mistaken perceptions
are wrong impressions that are mired
in false appearances.*

Viparyayo mithya jnyanam atadrupa prathistham.

In between hundreds or thousands of correct perceptions, we might miss-see something completely. I'm driving down the road at dusk on a windy autumn day, and a small mouse scurries across the road under my tires. I slam on the brakes with a screech.

Then I realize that the "mouse" was only the false appearance of a mouse: it was really only a dry leaf blown across the road. And then there's this momentary sense of emptiness—the mouse is gone, it was never there—followed by a slightly foolish feeling as I continue down the road.

Now it's absolutely essential to realize that, on one level, even our correct perceptions are all incorrect. That is, the socks in my hand are socks—that's correct. But deep in my heart is this belief that they are socks that are in my hand because I own them, because I found them at the store, and because I bought them.

All of *these* ideas about my socks are completely incorrect. There are no socks like that—no more than the man in the movie. It's all the Great Mistake, a mistaken perception that causes all the pain in the world.

9 Pictures in the Mind

*I.9–11 Imagination is a mental impression
that follows a word,
and is devoid of any concrete basis.
Sleep is a case where the mind turns
without any object at all
to help it grow.
Memory is the ability not to forget
an object that you have experienced.*

*Shabda jnyaya-anupati vastu shunyo vikalpah.
Abhava pratyaya vishaya-asampramoshah smirtih.*

When we plan a dinner, we see in our minds the finished meal, although that meal doesn't yet correspond to any concrete thing. The words "What's for dinner?" inspire this picture in our imagination.

Most of our perceptions during the day are triggered by some outside object: seeing an apple is set off by the apple—in a sense the seeing depends, or hinges upon, the apple. When we sleep or dream there may not be any such outer object, but still the mind is turning, or operating, at a low level.

When we have a memory of something, again there is no outer object: just an approximate picture in the mind, sort of a shorthand note to remind us of something.

And so in the course of an entire day, our mind wends its way through different outside objects and inside images or thoughts. But unless we truly understand things—unless we understand what yoga really means—then every single perception and imagination we ever have is infected by the Great Mistake. Feelings, strong feelings, come up about the things we think we see—and the child beats her fist against the bad man on the screen.

10 Approaching the Door

I.12–13 Stopping it requires constant practice,
and giving up your attachments.
Constant practice means
striving to be there.

Abhyasa vairagyabhyam tan nirodhah.
Tatra sthitau yatnobhyasah.

The way to stop the Great Mistake is to work our way through all five of the paths. We reach the first path by giving up our attachments, and this requires developing the habit of constant practice.

In a general sense, "constant practice" here means the willingness to work very hard to reach our perfect destiny, far beyond the mistakes our mind now makes. Quite simply, we will never be able to complete all the hard work needed to reach our destiny if we don't have a very strong motivation for doing so.

This motivation comes to all of us at some point in our lives. Most often it is some kind of personal disaster or tragedy: the person we most love dies or leaves us, we find out we have cancer—anything that wakes us up to what really matters. People are in pain, and it's up to us to help them. It is our destiny to be the one who helps them.

We begin with a daily inner practice. It will always include three essential elements: being careful never to hurt others; learning to pray or meditate; and relentlessly exploring the question of where things really came from.

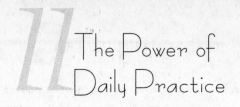

The Power of Daily Practice

*I.14 You must cultivate your practice
over an extended period of time;
it must be steady, without gaps,
and it must be done correctly—
for then a firm foundation is laid.*

*Sa tu dirgha kala nairantarya
satkara-asevito dirdha bhumih.*

Changing the mind, the heart, is infinitely more difficult than anything else we do—more demanding than education or work or rais-
ing a family. It takes time, and we need to give it that time, for as
long as it takes.

And the time must be given daily: our spiritual practice must become a regular part of our day, as important as eating or working or
sleeping. Our minds are infinitely powerful. We can learn to be good
at anything, if only we give it an hour or two of practice a day. But
every day.

We all know that there are right ways of fixing a car and wrong
ways too. If you try to fix your car but you don't know what you are
doing, you can really make expensive mistakes.

Fixing heart and mind are no different. We need to know what
we're doing—we need good, clear instructions on what to do, from
someone who's already done it.

Learning how to maintain a really effective daily practice creates
a perfect foundation for entering the first of the five paths.

12 Attachment to Distraction

I.15 Giving up your attachments
consists of the decision to gain control
over your craving for experiences,
seen or only heard of.

Drishta-anushravika vishaya vitirshnasya
vashikara sanjnya vairagyam.

It is our destiny, each one of us, to save the world. Yes, we can, and
we will. Deep inside of us we know this is what we want to do, and
why we came to this world in the first place. On some level we dream
of this all the time; it is why almost all the novels and movies created
by our culture have a heroine or hero who saves the day. Because we
ourselves want to. We need to.

And so we step onto the first of the five paths. It's called the Path
of Accumulation—piling up enough goodness, enough power, to
change ourselves and our world. We take this step by deciding that
we can no longer bear the pain all around us.

Now we will no longer have any time for the meaningless distractions of life—we must simplify our lives, concentrate on what's
really important. No more time to only work and eat and sleep and
die—no more time to waste on newspapers and television to hear
about how others wasted their time.

13 Attachment to Illusion

1.16 In its highest form, it is the freedom from attachment to solid things, gained by one to whom the true nature of the person has been revealed.

Tat param purusha khyater guna vaitirshnyam.

When we take a trip by airplane, we tend to focus on small things: the food, the movie, the person next to us.

Then if the plane suddenly drops, we forget all the small things. We think about death, about what we did with our life, about what might happen after we die.

But we can (and will) die any time, even sitting in a chair at home. The plane is always dropping. It's alright—it's a good thing—to enjoy life. We should enjoy it. But we should also enjoy the work of finding its deeper meaning, and not lose our life in little distractions and attachments.

The worst attachment of all is to be attached to the idea that the things all around us exist out there on their own, concretely, in the sense that they don't depend on how we lead our lives.

We begin to see through this wrong idea when we reach the second path: the Path of Preparation. Here we begin to realize—if only intellectually—that our own true nature, and the nature of everything else in the world, is that we very much come from how we treat others.

14 Meditation Traps

*I.17 Noting, examining, deep pleasure,
and being in oneself are still the type
done consciously, for they lead to that of form.*

*Vitarka vichara-ananda-asmita
rupa-anugamat samprajnyatah.*

At the Path of Preparation, we begin serious meditation to try to see the way things really are. Our culture is new to the art of meditation; there are hundreds of different kinds, and some of them are just a temporary escape.

Meditation is a serious tool. We need to use it to fix ourselves and the world, forever. Using meditation only to feel good for a while is like a surgeon taking the anesthesia himself, leaving the patient to die on the operating table.

There are four types of meditation that can lead us, after we die, to a useless place called the Realm of Form. Some of these same meditations, if practiced without a conscious mental state that is infected by the Great Mistake, can save your life. You need to learn the difference, from a qualified teacher.

Moving up through these four types of meditation is similar to listening to your favorite song. At first you only note that the song is being played. Then you begin to examine the beauty of the words and melody. A feeling of deep pleasure washes over you, and finally you go beyond even the pleasure, losing yourself in the song completely.

15

Bombs that Never Explode

I.18–19 That type where you still have
unripe seeds, but where
—because of your previous practice—
the factor is suppressed,
is the other kind.
Those who stay in that nature,
in the factor of becoming,
take the same gross physical body.

Virama pratyaya-abhyasa purvah
sanskara sheshonya.
Bhava pratyaya videha prakirti layanam.

We have billions upon billions of seeds in our minds, planted there by hurting or taking care of those around us. When the time is right, individual seeds sprout up in our minds at about the speed of the individual frames in a movie, and we watch the stream of our life unfold.

The seeds that are still waiting to sprout are called "unripe" seeds. The factor that makes harmful seeds sprout is simply seeing things the wrong way. When we practice well—that is, when we learn how to avoid meditation traps and use our meditation in this other way, the right way—then we can keep bad seeds from ever sprouting.

Death itself comes from a bad seed sprouting. The body only gets old because bad seeds are sprouting. Herein lies the secret of the water of life.

When bad seeds are about to sprout, we call it "becoming." This is triggered by staying in our same old nature or state, seeing things the wrong way. These seeds are what gave us a mortal body in the first place, and we can change that—if we change the seeds.

16 The Five Powers

I.20 The other ones must first use belief, effort, awareness, meditation, and wisdom.

Shraddha virya smirti samadhi prajnya purvaka itaresham.

We want to be people who follow the "other kind" of meditation and practice—the ones who go beyond a body of flesh and blood. To do this, we need to learn the Five Powers: five different spiritual skills that speed us along the Path of Preparation.

The first power is belief. This is not blind faith, but rather a deep attraction for the beauties of spiritual life, once we have heard about them and understand we can reach them ourselves. Effort then comes naturally: once you know what a chocolate-chip cookie tastes like, you're naturally willing to go through some work to get one. Spiritual effort in gladness is doing good things for others.

On one level, awareness is to be present: to be here now, not wrapped up in what's happened or might happen. On another level, it is watching that whatever we do or say or think is something noble.

The highest form of awareness is to keep our mind on where the things that happen to us are really coming from. Meditation here is the ability to stay in deep thoughts on this question; and asking the question within this meditation is itself wisdom.

The Four Stages

I.21–22 The goal is reached by those who act with intense dedication and urgency. There is, furthermore, a distinction of lesser, medium, and highest.

Tivra samveganam asannah.
Mirdu madhya-adhimatratvat
tatopi visheshah.

If a young child falls into a fire, her mother moves quickly. People having a normal life in this world are in much more danger than the child. On the Path of Preparation, we pass through four stages that prepare us for the next path, the all-important Path of Seeing. These four steps are called Warmth, Peak, Mastery, and the Highest Object of All. Our five spiritual skills develop to a higher degree at each stage, turning from the Five Powers into the Five Peaks, then the Five Strengths, and finally the Five Highest Objects.

The four stages represent a growing realization of the Great Mistake—a growing understanding of where things are really coming from. The stages begin with an appreciation of how objects in the world around us might be coming from ourselves. They end when we turn this understanding inside, upon our own minds.

A person at the end of the fourth stage might be standing, watching a pot of water on the stove. He suddenly realizes that he is only watching an impossibly perfect, tiny picture of a pot within his own mind. Eyes after all don't think; they can only see some silver-colored circle.

18 The Master

I.23–24 And another way
is to ask the Master
for her blessing.
A master is an extraordinary person
who is untouched by mental afflictions,
by deeds, their ripening, and their storing.

Ishvara pranidhanad va.
Klesha karma vipaka-ashayair
aparamirshtah purusha
vishesha ishvara.

It can take a very long time to develop the Five Powers to the point of the pot on the stove. Another way is simply to seek the extraordinary power that comes from direct contact with a Master—a living person who has experienced these things directly, and can teach them to us.

There are things we absolutely cannot learn from the dead pages of a book, or the wires of a computer.

Finding our own personal Master is something we absolutely need to do. It's an art in itself; take your time. Look for a person who really understands where things are coming from. This will make them a gentle, noble person, since this understanding is the only thing that can stop negative thoughts like anger forever.

No anger, no hurting others. No hurting, no new bad seeds in the mind. And understanding itself means that bombs stored up in the mind earlier will now simply never explode.

Look then for a Master who understands.

19 Serving

I.25–26 Herein lies,
in the most excellent way of all,
the seed for knowing all things.
This teacher is one as well
whom those of days gone by
never allowed themselves to be separated from,
for any length of time.

Tatra niratishayam sarvajnya bijam.
Sa purvesham api guruh
kalena-anavachedat.

The things around us are a product of the seeds within our own minds. And so are the people. In a sense then we make our own spiritual Master.

It's a kind of magic that happens when we find a truly qualified teacher and then have the opportunity to serve her. No blind faith here either: with our eyes wide open; having checked the person first, carefully; aware of human weaknesses (and how those we see in others come too from ourselves), we commit ourselves to the joy of working closely with a spiritual guide, and serving her and her sacred work. There is no greater way to plant the seed for ourselves to become a perfect, enlightened being who can truly help all beings.

The bond between us and our spiritual guide is the sweetest and most meaningful relationship we will ever enjoy. Ultimately it will help countless people. For this reason too it can attract great obstacles: the more powerful the good, the more powerful the negative forces attracted to it.

Stay as close as you can to your Master, and to the friends you have who are good people. Goodness rubs off on us.

20 The Highest of Prayers

I.27–29 Calling upon them
is the first of all prayers.
You must repeat this prayer,
and think well upon its meaning.
With this you will gain the ability
to focus the mind within,
and to avoid all obstacles.

Tasya vachakah pranavah.
Taj japas tad artha bhavanam.
Tatah pratyak chetana-
adhigamopyantaraya-abhavash cha.

These lines are about mantra. A mantra is a short, essential prayer that makes wishes come true. Mantras only work if two requirements are fulfilled: the mantra must have come from a truly holy person, and the person saying it must be someone who is truly kind to others.

There are countless kinds of mantras or prayers. The very highest prayer is simply to call upon your own Master for help. Even just calling his name, quietly, to yourself throughout the day is enough, if your mind is focused upon how your teacher will help you learn to help others.

Repeating this Master Prayer keeps the mind focused within and less wrapped up in the outside world. Because of the extraordinary power that comes when a spiritual teacher and a spiritual student honor and serve each other purely, all obstacles in your life will melt away.

If you wish, you can add the word "Om" before your Master's name when you repeat it. This sacred sound is made of three parts, which represent the totally pure actions and words and thoughts you will use to help others reach the end of the five paths.

21 Beginning Obstacles

I.30a Obstacles occur when the mind is distracted,
and this can be caused by illness, fogginess in the mind,
having doubts, carelessness, and laziness . . .

Vyadhi 'styana sanshaya pramada-alasya
avirati bhranti darshana-alabdha
bhumikatva-anavasthitatvani
chitta vikshepas tentarayah.

We have too much to do, too much to think about. It's all our own choice, but it gets worse under certain conditions. Here begins a list of major obstacles to the life of the spirit.

Illness is obviously an obstacle but can also become a fulfilling spiritual practice. It inspires us to work on what's really important in life, and makes us more humble and sympathetic of others who have problems.

Mental fogginess or dullness comes for example from not enough sleep, or too much food. As a culture we have perfected gluttony and abolished the word. It keeps our minds from operating quickly and clearly.

Incorrect meditation can also leave us a little foggy-headed. Real meditation gives us a bright, clear, strong mind that enables us to do anything well, from dishes to computers to ultimate reality.

Examining spiritual ideas critically is excellent; doubt in the form of avoiding the job of figuring out life is not. Carelessness here is not staying aware of how our actions affect others and ourselves—alcohol and drugs are ideal ways to cultivate carelessness. Laziness is when we simply don't feel like doing things that we know are good and helpful for everyone.

22 Ultimate Obstacles

I.30b . . . And by mistaken views of the world
that are left uncorrected,
failing to reach specific levels,
or not being established in them firmly.

How we view the world—our worldview—is in the end the only thing that decides whether we suffer or find real happiness.

It's extremely important to realize that an entire civilization can be caught up for many years in a disastrously mistaken view of the world. For thousands of years sensible people believed that the world was flat. The courageous, democracy-minded founders of the United States kept human beings as slaves and believed they were animals, not people.

Our culture today has its own massively mistaken ideas of the world, and these cause all the hunger, poverty, sickness, and war in the world. If our people's view of the world is causing pain to others and ourselves, then we must look for a better one, one that works. If it doesn't work, we cannot simply continue to follow whatever we learned as children, whether it came from parents or schools, churches or governments. True yoga is the search for a worldview that actually works to bring people happiness.

There are specific levels in our path where we eliminate, forever, different spiritual obstacles like doubt. We need to learn what these levels are, how to reach them, and how to stay there.

23 Inner and Outer

I.31 The mind flies off,
and with that comes pain in the body;
unhappy thoughts; shaking in the hands
and other parts of your body;
the breath falling out of rhythm
as it passes in and out.

Duhkha daurmanasya angam ejayatva
shvasa prashvasa vikshepa sahabhuvah.

Yoga is also the union of the inner and outer methods for reaching total purity. This union depends upon the connection between our physical outer body and our spiritual inner body.

Our entire being is like the layers of an onion. The outermost layer is the gross physical body. The next layer down is what feeds this layer, the breath being our most important "food." This breath layer is linked to a layer of subtle physical energy called *prana*, or the "inner winds."

These winds flow throughout our body in the next layer, a network of tiny tubes or channels more subtle than the finest light. Upon the winds in these channels ride our thoughts themselves, the innermost layer, like a rider atop a horse: the amazing frontier where mind and body meet.

In a negative way, problems at one layer of this onion affect all the others. If our thoughts are unstable, this disturbs the inner winds upon which they ride. This then disturbs the breath, and causes nervousness and shaking.

This ultimately causes physical ailments like ulcers or heart problems, which again sets off unhappy thoughts—a continuous downward spiral. The outer exercises and inner meditations of yoga reverse this cycle.

24 The Four Infinite Thoughts

*I.32–33a And if you wish to stop these obstacles,
there is one, and only one,
crucial practice for doing so.
You must use kindness, compassion, joy, and equanimity.
Learn to keep your feelings in balance,
whether something feels good
or whether it hurts; whether something is enjoyable
or distasteful . . .*

*Tat pratisheda-artham eka tattva abhyasah.
Maitri karuna muditopekshanam sukha duhkha
punya-apunya vishayanam . . .*

There is one crucial practice for stopping all obstacles, and this is the Four Infinite Thoughts. They are called "infinite" because, in the end, we look upon infinite living creatures on infinite worlds with our own eyes, in a single moment, and love them all.

Infinite kindness is the desire to bring all living beings happiness. And it means deciding that I myself will make it happen, even if no one else wants to help me. Infinite compassion is the decision to remove the pain of every living being, by myself if need be.

Infinite joy is the decision to bring all living beings to a higher form of happiness. A cup of coffee or cocoa makes almost anyone happy. But we don't finish feeling happy until we can actually help and serve countless other people.

Infinite equanimity is the decision to help *everybody* this way—not just our friends or family. Equanimity begins with avoiding extremes of feelings: happy when we feel well, or not when we don't.

Which is only to say we shouldn't be thrown off balance by how we feel. We *must* of course escape all pain and achieve all happiness—and we must desire to do so.

25 Bright and Clear

I.33b–35 ... *This practice makes the mind*
bright and clear as pure water.
It gives the same effect as releasing,
then storing, the wind of the breath.
It also helps us control the tendency
that we have, of thoughts constantly arising
about outer objects of experience.

... *bhavanatash chitta prasadanam.*
Prachardana vidharanabhyam va pranasya.
Vishayavati va pravirttir utpanna
manasah sthiti nibhandani.

A daily meditation on the Four Infinite Thoughts changes our entire life. It gives our life real and lasting meaning. Eating, earning and spending money, working for a house that we will lose, the slow descent into weak old age and death are not what we were meant to do with our lives. Deep inside, we know that very clearly.

That's why it makes our minds feel bright and clear when we hear someone say that our real purpose in life is to help and serve others; and not with kinds of help that will themselves quickly be used up and disappear. We were all meant for more.

The physical yoga exercises, and the special breathing techniques that go with them, are meant to open up the subtle inner channels. But because the thoughts themselves travel in these channels, we can get the same results—a lot more quickly and easily—by simply *thinking* these highest four thoughts of all.

We rarely really think about what others around us want or need. When we do, we find that we are released from our constant, exhausting compulsion for the bigger and better—clothes, food, money, fame.

26 Freedom from Selfishness

I.36–37 It also makes your heart carefree,
and radiant like starlight.
And it frees your mind from wanting things.

Vishoka va jyotishmati.
Vita raga vishayam va chittam.

The Four Infinite Thoughts ultimately trigger infinite love. This love begins when I quite seriously believe, after much thought and training, that it *is* possible for any normal person to become someone who can assist countless people all at once.

For a time, even now, this love is just an idea. But it gets stronger, and one day it explodes into the direct experience of ultimate love.

This feels completely different from what we normally think of as love. In almost all people, the inner channels at the heart are tangled and blocked. At the first instant of ultimate love, the inner winds break free in crystal-colored light from the heart. Physical yoga was created to help this happen.

When it does, then for a brief time we can actually see the face of every living being, not just in our world but on countless planets. And in this moment we see as well that we will spend every hour of the rest of our life, and lives beyond this one, learning to go and take care of each one of these beings. We are freed forever from selfishness and forever from wanting anything less than this.

27 The Deeper Powers

*I.38–40 It moreover enables you to be conscious
in your dreamlife, as you sleep.
It brings you to the same exhilaration
as deep meditation does.
You gain mastery over the tiniest atoms,
and galaxies as well.*

Svapna nidra jnyana-alambanam va.
Yatha-abhimata dhyanad va.
Parama-anu parama mahattvantosya vashi kara.

We've talked about how our world is a product of the seeds within our own minds. Just *wanting* to help a single other person alters these seeds drastically. The wish to help infinite numbers of people—even if it is only a wish, and a very feeble wish at first—has the power to transform all the seeds within our minds. This then transforms—well—everything there is, everywhere.

Naturally this effect spreads to all those states of mind we go through in a normal day. The act of sleep itself becomes an adventure—we're as lucid in dreams as we are in our everyday life, and we use our sleeping hours to explore and improve both mind and heart.

If meditation can bring us a kind of bliss, then simply standing in the kitchen and thinking the four thoughts brings us the same bliss, with a lot less effort.

As the seeds in our mind transform, we suddenly become very good at anything we try to do—whether small exacting tasks or monumental projects. As this process continues, we even gain the power to actually enter and alter processes from subatomic to galactic levels—if that would help somebody.

28 Path of the Diamond

I.41 Those extraordinary people who shatter the way
the mind turns things around use a balanced meditation,
which is fixed and clear on its object.
And the object is like a crystal,
with the one that holds it, and what it holds,
and the holding itself as well.

Kshina virtter abhijatasyeva
maner grahitir girhana grahyeshu
tat stha tat anjanata samapattih.

The most important moment of our life is when we see ultimate reality for the first time at the third path, the Path of Seeing. It changes us forever, and brings us to the very verge of our goal.

This path cannot occur unless first we are staying in the state of meditation with a totally clear and focused mind: balanced, free of the two extremes of dullness and hyperactivity.

During this first brief period in ultimate reality we cannot perceive anything less than the ultimate. And so we are for a while like water poured into water, unaware of ourselves or even that we are seeing, for these are not the ultimate things that we are looking upon with our minds.

Ultimate reality is like a crystal; specifically, like a diamond, and we will know it is so. Nothing can be ultimate—highest or hottest—because we can always add another inch or degree. But the diamond comes close, for nothing else in the universe can scratch it.

Ultimate reality lies all around us now, but beyond our sight, clear as diamond. In fact everything there is, everywhere, possesses its own ultimate reality—just as every splinter of diamond is simple, perfect purity.

29 Remember What You Saw

I.42–43 When you grasp this with images,
mixing up the word and the object,
then that is the type of balanced meditation
which uses concepts.
Stay in that one pure thought, and never forget it;
that single most important thing: things are empty
of being what they are by themselves.
This is the clear light, beyond all conceptual thought.

Tatra shabda-artha jnyana vikalpaih
sankirna savitarka samapattih.
Smirti parishuddhau svarupa shunyeva-artha
matra nirbhasa nirvitarka.

We commune briefly with ultimate reality and then come down and back to our normal state of the Great Mistake, seeing things wrong. Except that now we *know* what we're doing wrong: we don't believe how we're seeing things, and thus there's the sense of an illusion going on.

At this point, the second step of the Path of Seeing, we must try to remember what we saw: that things are empty. This is the first time that the Master refers to emptiness.

Emptiness doesn't mean blackness, or that nothing exists, and certainly not that things like good and bad actions don't matter. It only means that what we thought was there isn't there—no more than a man on a movie screen. That is, if I look around and try to find anything that is *not* coming from seeds in my mind, I'll come up empty-handed: a simple absence, like colorless light.

Our minds in the Great Mistake mistake words—that is, the perfect little mental pictures that the seeds make—for actual objects. This in itself is thinking "conceptually" here. It's not that we want to stop thinking altogether!

30 Approaching the Goal

I.44–46 The distinction between what we refer to
as being "involved with examining"
or "not being involved with examining,"
moreover, has to do with the
relative subtlety of the object.
That object which is subtle to the ultimate
is the one where there are no signs.
And this is still what is called
"deep meditation where we still
have the seeds."

Etayaiva savichara nirvichara cha
sukshma vishaya vyakhyata.
Sukshma vishayatvam cha-alinga paryavasanam.
Ta eva sabijah samadhih.

So now we know that ultimate reality and emptiness and clear light and just that simple missing feeling when we find out there's no real man on the movie screen are all the same thing. The day after we see this directly, we are on the fourth path: the Path of Habituation.

It's called this because we are getting used to what we saw, using that indescribable experience to complete the work of removing negative seeds from our mind forever.

At this point we still have these seeds, even when we meditate, but we never again fall into those meditation traps that are just moving between subtle pleasant experiences: shifting mental gears lower and lower, beyond even examining the notes of the music, but with none of the *content* of meditation that can free us of the Great Mistake.

This *content* of our meditation, the object we use this powerful tool to focus upon, must be that one most meaningful and subtle object of all: the fact that the man on the screen simply isn't a man—all the "signs" of a man to him, real arms and legs and the like, disappear too when we touch the screen.

Beyond All Fear

*I.47–49 When you gain the fearlessness
of going beyond all examining, you reach inner bliss.
At that point, wisdom becomes vast and awakened.
You experience a completely different object
than with the wisdoms of hearing and reasoning,
because what you see is far beyond.*

*Nirvichara vaisharadyedhyatma prasadah.
Irtambhara tatra prajnya.
Shrutanumana prajnyabhyam anya
vishaya vishesha-arthatvat.*

As we travel along the Path of Habituation, we eliminate within our-selves, forever, all negative thoughts like anger, jealousy, or wanting things ignorantly. The last negative thought that we overcome is even the most subtle form of examining or seeing things the wrong way.

Once all negativity is gone, we progress through the final steps to total purity. This period is devoted to gaining the ability to see every-thing in the universe—whether past, present, or future—at the same time: a useful trick for helping others.

Our wisdom is not only vast, but also awakened.

Even very advanced people can only see ultimate reality during deep meditation, and at that time cannot experience things of nor-mal reality. When we reach total purity though we blissfully see everything in both realities, even with our ears and fingers and other senses. It's difficult for us to imagine.

This is the fifth path, the final goal, the Path of No More Learning. We are beyond all fear, and we're not afraid to announce it to the world. We have reached our goal through the careful process of learning from a Master and considering well what he says; now we experience it directly.

32 The End of the Seeds

I.50–51 The mental seed thus created
cuts off all other seeds.
And when mental seeds are stopped
in this way, everything is stopped;
Thus it is known as deep meditation
where we no longer have the seeds.

Taj-jah sanskaro-nya sanskara pratibandhi.
Tasya-api nirodhe sarva nirodhan
nirbijah samadhih.

Now we have new seeds that cut off all our old, negative seeds—both those that caused the Great Mistake and those that limited us from knowing all things.

One vast group of the new seeds creates a paradise around us, where we dwell forever with everything, and everyone, we ever hoped for. We enter this heaven whenever in our lives we reach this much goodness within ourselves, and we enter it wherever we are, without leaving or coming.

Another vast group of seeds acts spontaneously, without any conscious thought on our part, to send us out to billions of suffering beings. We appear at their side, in whatever way they need—as a pet dog, as a spiritual guide, as a lover, as an enemy to test their virtues.

We do all this without stirring from a perfectly still and pure state of being. We are perfect knowledge, which by merely being plants the seeds that make itself continue, eternally.

Second Cornerstone

The Chapter on the Way

Reaching to Reach

II. 1–2 Undertaking difficult spiritual practices,
regular study, and prayers to the Master
are ways of becoming whole
that are activities.
Now the whole purpose of meditation
is to make our negative thoughts
dwindle away.

Dvitiyah Sadhana Padah

Tapah svadhyayeshvara
pranidhanani kriya yogah.
Samadhi bhavana-artha
klesha tanu karana-arthash cha.

The second cornerstone upon which the house of yoga is built is the
Way. In the first chapter we use deep meditation to travel through
the five paths; in the second chapter we start some very practical yoga
methods to attain this meditation, and the wisdom that rides it. The
two chapters together reflect yoga as a union of inner, mental methods and outer, physical methods or activities.

It's important to be clear about where we want our yoga to take
us. What goal do we have in mind? The first important goal is nirvana. This is not some stupefied numbness, but refers rather to per-
manently stopping all our negative thoughts. Imagine yourself as a
person who is simply not capable of getting angry, ever again.

After reaching this nirvana, we work further to become a holy being—something like an angel really—who sees all things and helps
all people.

In fact, the Sanskrit word for "the Way" here is *sadhana*, which
means "to reach" angels through our steady, daily practice. We reach
them first by contacting them. We reach them secondly by *becoming*
them.

*II.3–4 The five negative thoughts are ignorance,
selfness, liking, disliking, and grasping.
Ignorance is the field for the ones
that come after it, whether they are
dormant, dwindling, interrupted, or flourishing.*

*Avidya-asmita raga
dvesha-abhiniveshah pancha kleshah.
Avidya kshetram uttaresham
prasupta tanu vichinnodaranam.*

The best way to get out of trouble is to figure out how we got there in the first place. If water is pouring all over the floor, you can either mop all day or simply turn off the tap.

There are four important principles that—when we grasp them totally—help stop all our pain. These are called the Four Higher Truths. Here we begin the first: the truth of where our pain comes from. The Master takes us step-by-step through the entire process of how we cause ourselves trouble.

At the very bottom of everything lies the fertile field of ignorance—what we've been calling the Great Mistake, or how the mind turns things around the wrong way. Only by stopping this ignorance can we stop all our other unhappiness, anger, and the rest.

Oh, we can try to get more sleep, or take a vacation, do a little yoga or light meditation to calm our harried minds. This doesn't stop thoughts like anger, it just suppresses or interrupts them for a while. Their root, the ignorance, is always still there. And as long as it is, the calm will wear off at the first big traffic jam.

35 The Four Mistakes

II.5 In ignorance we misunderstand our world:
things that cannot last,
things that are unclean, and painful,
and that are not themselves;
seem to us as if they will last,
and as if they are clean,
and pleasant, and very much themselves.

Anitya-ashuchi duhkha-anatmasu
nitya shuchi sukha-atma khyatir avidya.

If aliens came to our world from another planet, an enlightened planet, they would be shocked and saddened by how we live. Because we are completely wrong about everything we think is good.

Instead of trying to figure out where things really come from, instead of trying to find out why good things end, we simply and blindly work our lives away, to get things that we all know cannot and will not last. Houses, cars, positions, friends, families, death.

We spend billions of dollars on soaps and creams and cosmetics and clothes to drape over something that is already beginning to rot.

Our attempts to seek pleasure or rest are often only painful, and the few pleasures we do manage to obtain always end in pain.

These are ignorance, yes, but again at the bottom of them all is root ignorance: the fact that every single thing we ever see is not what we think it is. Things are not themselves—they are ourselves.

All living creatures, even ants, make this mistake about things. Ignorance at this first stage is a seed that lies within us, before we are even born.

36 The Beginning of Me

II.6 Selfness is where the wrong impression
of someone seeing something
and the something someone sees
make it seem as if
each one were itself.

Dirg darshana shaktyor
eka-atmateva-asmita.

So we enter life with the seed of ignorance within us. And then in the very womb the seed flowers into a personal experience of this misunderstanding, which is here called "selfness."

This wrong idea of "me" is awakened by our very first sensations in life: the warmth and pressure within our mother. Poisoned by ignorance, the mind immediately splits life into "warmth" and "me feeling the warmth."

It's very important to say here that there is a "me" that is perfectly fine—one that does exist, and that experiences other things. So what's the difference between this me and the one that causes all the trouble?

When we do experience an object like warmth, we tend to think of it as something out there, on its own, by itself. We tend to think that how it *got* out there in the first place was from something outside of ourselves: it comes from a fire, it comes from my mother's body.

But in fact the warmth, and me too for that matter, is being produced by those seeds within my own mind. We can see this from the fact that cozy warm for one person is stifling hot to another.

37 Is It Wrong to Like Things?

II. 7–9 Assailed by what feels good,
we begin to like things.
Assailed by what feels bad,
we begin to dislike things.
Grasping is a thought
that comes all on its own,
even for those who understand,
and then grows ever stronger.

Sukha-anushayi ragah.
Duhkha-anushayi dveshah.
Svarasa vahi vidushopi
tatha rudhobhiniveshah.

"Grasping" here means ignorance as it misunderstands an object in the moment. We enter a pastry shop and see a single maple-coated donut left on the tray.

Temporarily blinded by our feelings for maple-coated donuts, even those of us who to some extent *understand* the Great Mistake begin to grasp, despite ourselves. Grasping doesn't mean grabbing the donut, or even wanting it a lot. It just means looking at it the wrong way: It's out there, on the tray. It's there because someone baked it. I will get it because I have money. None of which is true.

Now it's not *wrong* to like donuts. Spiritually advanced people *enjoy* things like donuts a lot more than we can. The very *ability* to like and dislike is what gets us enlightened: I like peace, I don't like pain, I dislike seeing people suffer.

Heaven itself is bliss, not some place where yogis sit around trying not to enjoy anything. But there's a difference between *smart* liking and *stupid* liking. How do we tell them apart?

Here's a test. An elderly lady behind you says to her husband, "Maple's my favorite!" Do you like the donut enough to leave it for her?

38 Fixing the World

II.10–11 *Cutting off their flow*
requires the elimination
of very subtle problems.
These ways that the mind turns
are eliminated by deep meditation.

Te pratiprasava heyah sukshmah.
Dhyana heyas tad virttayah.

Back to the bad man on the movie screen. He's hurting a puppy. It's something I don't like.

The seed of ignorance triggers misunderstanding me and things, which triggers immediate blindness, which allows my mind to pose the following moral quandary:

Do I run up to the screen and hit the bad man? Or do I run up to the screen and try to talk him out of his violence peacefully?

Get it. It's not that one of these methods, as they stand, would work better than the other. My crazy mind has lured me into choosing between two false opposites. The point is that *neither* approach will work, because neither approach *could* ever work. *That* man's not the man!

If we don't like what we're seeing—and in fact it *is* something unpleasant—we obviously have to go up to the booth where the movie projector is and change something there. It's an infinitely more subtle approach, but we don't really have any choice. If we want to stop pain, we have to stop the seeds.

And this is done in the mind, in deep meditation, beginning with the seeds that cause the Great Mistake.

39 Where the World Comes From

II.12–13 *These negative thoughts*
are the very root of the storehouse,
planted by the things we do.
And then we experience things,
in lifetimes we see or not.
As long as this root is still there,
then we will experience the ripening
of these actions in our lives to come.

Klesha mulah karma ashayo
dirshta-adirshta janma vedaniyah.
Sati mule tad vipako
jatyayur bhogah.

So here I am at the last maple-coated donut. I see it as something I get from a store and some money, not from my own seeds. I want it in a way that's mistaken about how to get it.

And so rather than taking care to plant seeds for a donut (by leaving this one for the lady behind me), I force the issue. I take the last donut, and thereby do a "karma."

Our mind is like an extraordinarily sensitive video camera that records every act, word, and thought we ever undertake, every second of our entire life. The image of each action or karma is stored in the mind as a seed. When the time comes, the seed ripens and creates everything around us and inside us.

This storehouse of seeds decides what we see now and also what we see where we can't see yet: after we die. Don't be naïve and believe that thoughts stop just because the body stops. If you don't get a call from someone, it doesn't mean they're dead. Maybe their phone is just broken.

We all have lots of old bad seeds. Knowledge can stop them from ever growing.

40 Where Pain Comes From

II.14 There is a connection of cause and effect:
the seeds ripen into experiences
refreshingly pleasant or painful in their torment;
depending on whether you have done good to others,
or done them wrong instead.

Te hlada paritapa phalah
punya-apunya hetutvat.

Take a moment of total honesty and ask yourself where the pain in your life is coming from. There are basically three choices.

The first is the Big Bang Theory. All things, including your irritating boss, have been caused by an event that conveniently has no cause itself. Your life, and all its tragedies, is simply a huge coincidence, as random particles from a very old explosion bump into each other, creating the face of every person you've ever met.

Or else there is a higher and infinitely compassionate intelligence that has created everything, and created it in such a way that we always lose everything to the agonies of old age, cancer, war, death.

Or else we get exactly what we give to others: a sort of perfect cosmic justice, as unforgiving as gravity. Let go of the coffee cup, it falls and breaks. Hurt someone else, you get hurt back.

All this, by the way, is not to say that there are no divine beings hovering around us constantly, guiding us toward perfect happiness. There are. But it cannot come unless we take care of others.

Why Things Fall Apart

> *II.15 The torment of change is caused*
> *by those same seeds of suffering;*
> *and stopping how the mind turns things around*
> *to have qualities of their own*
> *allows us to discern how, truly,*
> *every part of our lives is suffering.*

Parinama tapa sanskara duhkhair
guna virtti virodhach cha
duhkham eva sarvam vivekinah.

You meet somebody new, somebody exciting, and the feeling is mutual. In six months you can't stand each other.

Why do things fall apart? It's not your fault, or theirs. It's a problem with the way life itself is designed. It's that seed thing again.

Meeting a new friend is, like everything else, the result of a seed ripening within our own mind. Every minute that we spend with our new friend, this seed is wearing out, simply by producing our friend.

As the seed wears out, the relationship changes. When the seed sputters to an end, so does the friendship. When we understand how seeds work, we stop misunderstanding friends. They are not friends out there, who themselves have a smile or a touch that we enjoy. Everything is coming from the seeds.

Everything comes from the seeds, and seeds die by being born. Truly, then, every part of our lives—even the good things—must one day cause us pain. This is the second higher truth: the truth of pain.

42 Why Good People Suffer

*II.16 The pain that we
are ridding ourselves of
is all the pain
that would have come to us
in the future.*

Heyam duhkam anagatam.

If everything we ever experience is a result of how we treat others, then why do good people suffer? And why do people who cheat get rich?

It's crucial to realize that mental seeds act just like physical seeds. No one puts a corn seed into the ground and then stands there, expecting corn to pop up in a day or two.

Mental seeds are planted in the mind *simply by our being aware that we are doing, or saying, or thinking something toward someone else*. Seeds enter the storehouse and wait to be called up, like airplanes standing in line to take off.

Certain seeds, like priority flights, get to move ahead of the others in line; for example, if we have said something out of terrible anger, or done a kind deed with an intense understanding of how seeds themselves work.

In any case, it takes some time for the ripening process. It's very good to keep this in mind, since the time lag is deceiving and we can get discouraged. In actuality, anything good we ever do *always* comes back good. As does bad. When it seems differently, that's just an older seed taking off in between.

Everything We See

II.17–18 *The cause to be eliminated*
is the interaction between the seer
and what the seer sees.
And what we see, what appears to us,
is the state of all things:
they are either working or standing—
ourselves, a combination
of the elements and the powers;
something to consume, or to use
for our liberation.

Drashtir dirshyayo sanyogo heya hetuh.
Prakasha kriya sthiti shilam
bhutendriya-atmakam
bhoga-apavarga-artham dirshyam.

Here begins the third higher truth: the truth of the path to the end of pain. Let's take a glance at the way the universe itself is organized, and look for clues on how to stop the Great Mistake, the cause of all pain.

Everything we see around us is either at work or at rest. Things that work, or do something, change thereby. A few things, like the empty space or place that things stand in, never change.

We ourselves are ever-changing, a combination of physical elements like chemicals and conscious components such as our mind and powers of sense.

It's important to grasp that our perceptions of all things, whether they themselves are constant or in flux, are coming from the seeds in our minds. Then we can relate to the universe wisely. We can either blindly consume what our past seeds provide us, or embrace the bold endeavor of planting new seeds for a perfect world of freedom.

44 The Two Realities

II. 19–20 The phases that things exhibit
are the following:
differentiated, undifferentiated,
mere signs, or beyond all signs.
The seer, simply by seeing,
experiences purity;
but then later again sees objects.

Vishesha-avishesha linga matra
alingani guna parvani.
Drashta dirshi matrah
shuddhopi pratyaya-anupashya.

Another, very useful way of dividing up the universe is into the two realities. The first is called "deceptive reality": everything in our normal life, like donuts that look like you get them by paying.

Things in this lower reality seem different from each other, in and of themselves. A salad is not a donut. I am not you. We are innately and by definition *different*.

The second, higher reality we call "ultimate reality." On this level, a salad and a donut are not different. This is not some vague sentiment that everything is one; it's not, and we can't get anywhere with that. Rather, all things are *one* thing in that they come from our seeds. Now if we know this, we can build a new world, without pain.

Earlier on we caught our mind imposing a perfect little picture of a pot onto the mere signs of a pot out there on the stove: silver color, round shape. But even the silver is a picture imposed on two patches of silver, left and right.

When we understand thus how deceptive reality works, it leads us to see pure, ultimate reality; but we can't stay there without the right seeds.

45 The Loneliness of Seeing

II.21–22 This thing belongs only
to a person who has seen.
What is destroyed for one
who has reached this goal
is not, however, destroyed for others—
for they still possess the foundation.

Tad artha eva dirshyasya-atma.
Kirta-artha prati nashtam apyanashtam tad
anya sa-adharanatvat.

Only a person who has seen ultimate reality directly, on the Path of Seeing, truly understands the two realities. The experience is called "indescribable," only because the seer cannot convey it to another person in words that can make that person see it, on the spot. But of course a seer devotes the rest of his life to helping others see ultimate reality too.

And this is because the simple act of seeing, if only for a number of minutes, destroys certain negative emotions immediately—and all others not long afterward, bringing the freedom that all of us so desperately need.

In the hours after you first see, you pass through a series of extraordinary visions. One of these is seeing directly into the future, to the day when you will become a being of light who helps all other living creatures. And so all doubts about your future, for example, vanish forever.

These two are very personal experiences that can never be fully conveyed to those who have not seen. However much the seer may want to share them, however much he may say or write, he cannot remove every last doubt of those who have yet to shatter the Great Mistake.

46 Who's in Control?

II.23–25 *The cause of this, the interaction,*
is a state of mind that perceives
some real nature, due to a belief
in a master and servant.
And its cause is the misunderstanding.
When that is stopped, the interaction is stopped:
it is destroyed for one who sees,
as she reaches absolute purity.

Sva svami shaktyoh
svarupopalabdhi hetuh sanyogah.
Tasya hetur avidya.
Tad abhavat sanyoga-abhavo
hanam tad dirsheh kaivalyam.

Again, the reason that negative emotions must always continue in a person who has not seen is the way she feels that the things around them are separate from her, in the sense of not *coming* from them.

At the root of this misunderstanding lies the seed of ignorance, which we carried with us into this life. We said that seeing stops some negative thoughts immediately, and all others in time, inexorably, just because you saw.

The last negative thought to go is the Great Mistake, and all of its seeds. This is how seeing sends us toward the final goal, of absolute purity.

Want to know if you're still seeing things the wrong way? Look at the clothes you have on right now. Do you *own* them? Yes. Why? Because you control them. Oh, so can you tell me with certainty that you will own them tomorrow? Or may your family be dropping them off at the thrift shop, on the way to your funeral?

We don't own anything, not even our own body. It is no servant of ours, and we are not its master. No one is in control who has not yet seen.

47 To See the Illusion

II.26–27 People possessed of discrimination
that comes from the revelation
are no longer at a loss:
they now have a method
to accomplish this destruction.
Theirs is the wisdom
that carries one up
to the end of the seventh level.

Viveka khyatir aviplava hanopayah.
Tasya saptadha pranta bhumih prajnya.

And so we relate to the objects around us as though we owned them: as though we could control them in the moment, oblivious to the fact that we are completely at the mercy of whatever seeds we have planted in the past. Completely at the mercy of how we have treated others.

Seers don't relate to the world this way. During the period after their initial revelation—during the fourth path—those ancient, powerful seeds of ignorance in their minds still make the things around them seem as if they are happening *to* them and not *from* them.

But seers now *know* that they can't really be that way. And so, in a way, they see the illusion for what it is—even if they can't stop it yet.

Seers, because they have seen, possess all the tools they need to destroy all of the Great Mistake. Like a boat, this knowledge carries them through six advanced levels, where they perfect the virtues of giving, ethical living, patience, spiritual effort, deep meditation, and higher wisdom. During the seventh level, they manage to stop things from even *looking* like they come from their own side.

48 The Eight Limbs

II.28–29 If you engage earnestly in the various practices
of making yourself whole,
all your impurities will be destroyed;
and then you will gain the light of wisdom,
a revelation beyond even discrimination.
The eight limbs are self-control, commitments,
the physical poses, control of the breath,
withdrawal of the senses,
focus, fixation, and perfect meditation.

Yoga-anga-anushthanad ashuddhi kshaye
jnyana diptir aviveka khyateh.
Yama niyama-asana pranayama pratyahara
dharana dhyana samadhayoshtava-angani.

For seven higher levels, then, we see the illusion as an illusion, and finally stop things from even looking other than they really are: coming from our own seeds. We then embark on three final stages known as the "pure levels," where we learn to know all things, and to send ourselves out to guide people in many places at once.

Our wisdom here is beyond needing to stay mindful even of the illusion. This then is the fourth and final higher truth: the truth of the end of pain.

The brilliance of Master Patanjali's short book on yoga, the reason it has survived over thousands of years, is that it now gives us a very practical, step-by-step program that all of us—regardless of our abilities or the circumstances we live in—can undertake right now to gain these high goals.

We now begin these steps: the famous *ashta-anga*, the eight limbs or parts of the yoga path. As mentioned in the opening line of this second chapter, we cover first the five more externally oriented practices, concrete activities where our progress is easy to measure. These prepare us for the three more inwardly focused practices of the third chapter.

49 Self-Control

II.30a The different forms of self-control
are avoiding harm to anyone,
always telling the truth,
never stealing from another . . .

Ahinsa satya-asteya . . .

The first of the eight limbs of yoga is self-control, the ability in a sense to restrain ourselves from our more natural, lower instincts. Only the five most crucial forms of self-control are given.

The first is simply to avoid hurting other people; and remember that in the ancient books of wisdom, "people" means any living creature, however small or apparently unintelligent, since obviously they all feel pain and seek to avoid it.

The most serious form of hurting is to kill or cooperate in the killing of a human being. All of the ancient texts also state that a human being begins at conception, as consciousness enters the just-combined sperm and egg.

Really speaking the truth is difficult: it means never giving someone else even a slightly different impression from what you know to be true. The most serious lie is to make false claims about our spiritual realizations. It's also just generally good to avoid divisive talk, harsh words, and idle pratter.

Stealing is to take or use other people's property without their permission, which includes sneaking phone calls at work; dirtying up the city that we all pay for with our taxes; or ruining the earth for coming generations.

50 A Code for All of Us

II.30b–31 ... *Keeping sexual purity,*
and overcoming possessiveness.
These forms of self-control are mighty codes of conduct
meant for people at every stage of their personal development.
They go beyond differences in race or social status;
they go beyond the borders between countries;
they go beyond what is modern, or old;
they go beyond the various creeds and convictions.

... Brahmacharya-aparigraha yamah.
Jati desha kala samaya-anavachinnah
sarva bhauma mahavratam.

Sexual purity, for a person who has made a commitment to remain celibate, means avoiding all forms of sexual activity. When joyfully taken on and maintained, this vow grants extraordinary energy and mental clarity. For others, sexual purity means to strictly honor the bond between two other people who are in a committed relationship.

Avoiding possessiveness begins with making a determined effort to live simply. It also extends to recognizing and trying to stop our very common, very unfortunate feelings of displeasure when others get something nice, or our strange sense of satisfaction over others' problems.

These different forms of self-control are not an effort by some organization somewhere to keep us from having fun. The world is a messed-up place. The ultimate form of self-control is to stop thinking that this is someone else's fault: we create it with our own seeds. Avoiding actions that make bad seeds and a bad world is simply a smart thing for us to do.

It's not at all a matter of what religion or race or nation we belong to. Wise people throughout the history of our planet, in every country, have recognized that controlling ourselves is what truly sets us free.

51 Commitments

*II.32 The commitments are to be clean,
to be contented with whatever we have,
to embrace hardships for higher goals,
to engage in regular study,
and to seek our Master's blessings.*

*Saucha santosha tapah
svadhyayeshvara pranidhanani
niyamah.*

Five commitments make up the second limb of yoga. Self-control prevents bad seeds; the commitments plant good ones. These then actually create our success in the six other practices to come.

Keeping clean means striving all day to see that the world and all those around us are sacred. It also means not cluttering up our day with busyness, the craving for countless shallow interactions with others, and piles of completely meaningless junk lying around the temple of our home.

Contentment is not wanting the things that we don't have and enjoying the things that we do have. Yogis never complain about whatever food or place they may happen to get.

But contentment doesn't apply to our spiritual progress. We must be committed to finishing whatever hard work we need to, if it means taking ourselves and others forever out of pain. Regular study, in the old days, meant learning and memorizing the great books at the feet of a true Master. Our relationship with this Master is the greatest commitment of all, for without it we can never drink of the living water passed down from heart to heart, over thousands of generations of teachers and their students.

Destroying Old Bad Karma

II.33–34a When the images start to hurt you,
sit down and work out the antidote.
The images—people who hurt me or the like—
come from what I did myself;
or got others to do for me;
or what I was glad to hear that others had done.
And what came before them
was either craving, or hating, or dark ignorance.

Vitarka badhane pratipaksha bhavanam.
Vitarka hinsa-adayah
kirta karita-anumodita
lobha krodha moha purvaka . . .

So self-control and commitments stop new bad seeds and plant new good seeds. But we must also deal with the old bad seeds, stocked in our mental storehouse. Otherwise they will create obstacles for the other six practices of yoga.

We may not be able to see what we originally did to plant the seeds we have now, but we can decide what we must have done, from how these seeds are sprouting and creating painful pictures in our current health and relationships. This knowledge allows us to actually go in and destroy those seeds, within our own mind.

Seeds are planted not only by what we ourselves do, but also when someone else acts on our behalf; or simply if we consciously approve of an action. If a person dies in a war, and we have willingly paid taxes for that war, then the seed is the same as if we ourselves had plunged a knife into the person's chest, with our own hands.

All seeds for suffering—whether outright pain or happiness that decays into pain—are planted through the Great Mistake, as we respond to the events and people around us with mistaken feelings of liking and disliking things that actually come from ourselves.

53 The Four Forces

II.34b *They are of lesser, or medium,*
or greater power.
Say to yourself then,
"Who knows what pain
I have planted for myself?"
Sit down and work out the antidote.

. . . *Mirdu madhya adhimatra*
duhka-ajnyana-ananta phala iti
pratipaksha bhavanam.

There is a way to stop old bad karma. Otherwise things would be hopeless, since mental seeds constantly multiply in strength. A single acorn produces an oak tree weighing thousands of pounds, and mental seeds are no different.

Identify the most powerful negative seeds you have. Older ones that are causing a serious pain in your body. Newer ones that you remember planting: a particularly serious harm to someone; something done in extreme emotion; an injury to a powerful karmic object such as a parent or teacher.

The antidote has four steps: the Four Forces. Sit down first, and quietly review all you understand about seeds. Think about your destiny; simply, saving the world.

Second, feel some intelligent regret—not guilt—about how this action and its seed will delay your destiny.

The third and by far most important step is to decide not to repeat the mistake. For a health or relationship problem, you obviously need to strictly avoid any harm to others' well-being or friendships—and so on.

The fourth force is to take a positive action to counteract the negative one. Volunteer some time at a hospital, for example. Consciously dedicate all four forces to the seed, and it will die.

II.35 *If you make it a way of life*
never to hurt others,
then in your presence
all conflict comes to an end.

Ahinsa pratishthayam
tat sannidhau vaira tyagah.

What happens if we get good at managing our mental seeds? Remember first that only *we* can plant our own karmic seeds, and only *we* experience them when they sprout. (We can also do a good thing though as a group, and each person in that group plants a similar seed; this accounts for the prosperity and poverty that exist on opposite sides of our imaginary international borders.)

And so the Master says that "in *your* presence," something good will happen. And that's why two people can experience the very same yoga class as either an exhilarating adventure or just a very sore neck.

The more thoughtful and steadily we work with our own seeds instead of trying to wrestle with bad men on a movie screen, the more obvious it becomes that now we are on the right track.

The first stage is the *surprising*: a person who's a problem at work greets you warmly. Then the *obvious*: almost everybody at work starts to smile at you. Next, the *amazing*: wars around the world suddenly end. Finally, the *miraculous*: the process of your body aging clearly stops, and begins to reverse itself.

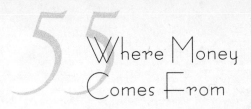

Where Money Comes From

*II.36–37 If you make it a way of life
always to tell the truth,
then anything you undertake
will have a successful result.
If you make it a way of life
never to steal from another,
then there will come a time
when people just come to you
and offer you all the money you need.*

Satya pratishthayam
kriya phala shrayatvam.
Asteya pratishthayam
sarva ratnopasthanam.

We have to get out of the mind-set that says telling a lie is only wrong if there's a good chance you can get caught at it. Or that it's only wrong because our parents said so, or our teachers at school, or because some religion says so.

The more we begin to understand seeds, the more clear it becomes that doing good things is not just right, but also the only way to get what we want—including what we want for everyone else.

If we work hard at telling the truth, then everyone else begins to be honest with us too, all the time. (Yet *please remember* the time gap: seeds need time to ripen, although the sheer understanding of how seeds work speeds this up wildly.) And then anything we ever undertake—be it a new business, a new relationship—just "automatically" works out.

Money karma can be amazing. Money isn't made at a federal facility somewhere. The *value* of the world economy—every single cent of it—is created by respecting other people's things. Give it a serious, prolonged try. You'll be laughing all the way to the bank.

56 How to Succeed in Relationships

> *II.38–39 If you make it a way of life*
> *always to keep sexual purity,*
> *then you will always have strength.*
> *If you persevere*
> *in overcoming possessiveness,*
> *you will be able to see*
> *your other lifetimes.*

Brahmacharya pratishthayam
virya labhah.
Aparigraha sthairye janma
katha-anta sambodhah.

It's no surprise that, karmically speaking (which is the only way that works anyway), we can get the kind of relationship we want with someone of the opposite sex only by being very careful not to damage other people's relationships.

A simple rule of thumb is always to act around another person's partner as if that other person were standing there too. Again, this is not a matter of what we normally think of as "morality": it's simply the only way that we can ever find a beautiful relationship ourselves; and if everyone acted this way, then *everyone* would have an amazing partner.

It's like respecting other people's things: if *everyone* understood it, then *everyone* in the world would have all they need. Poverty would be forever eradicated—and this is the only way it will ever occur.

The Sanskrit word for "strength" here implies both very good health in general and also a clean personal sexual vigor that gives you energy for everything you do.

If we learn not to clutter up our lives with things and busyness, the mind becomes so still and clear that we can see future events and even other lifetimes. A wonderful skill for success at every level of life!

Simply Clean

*II.40–41 If you stay clean,
then you will never find yourself
in crowds of the filthy.
Truth, purity, sweet thoughts,
single-pointedness, and
mastery of one's senses
are all qualities that make you
suitable for seeing
your true self.*

*Shauchat svanga
jugupsa parair asansargah.
Sattva shuddhi
saumanasyaikagryendriya
jaya-atma darshana
yogyatvani cha.*

If you continue to be very honest with yourself about the amount of pain that's really going on around us all the time, then the simple act of walking down a busy street can be overwhelming: hundreds of helpless, soon-to-be corpses brushing past us in a single hour.

If though we maintain a clean and sincere spiritual practice, then the habit of watching out for possible angels among us graduates into direct encounters with these beings. And angels really do exist: the idea may seem a little corny, but all the paintings and descriptions of them around attest to the fact that someone, somewhere, has actually met them.

If the seed thing really works, and if you push it to its limit, then it stands to reason that eventually you'll be surrounded by such beings, all the time.

Mental purity and physical simplicity lead to a serene state of mind, no longer enslaved by excesses of food or sex. When the water of a lake is perfectly still, only then can we see the full moon reflected in it: ultimate reality, emptiness.

58 How to Be Happy

II.42–43 *If you stay contented,
then you achieve
happiness that is unsurpassed.
Embracing spiritual hardships
destroys your impurities,
allowing you to master
both body and senses.*

*Santoshad anuttamah sukha labhah.
Kayendriya siddhir ashuddhi
kshayat tapasah.*

Want to get rich? It's easy. Simply purposefully collect the necessary karmic seeds to see yourself that way, and you *will* be. And so, paradoxically it seems, the only way to get a lot of money is to give a lot away, very purposefully and carefully.

But when the seeds ripen and it all comes back to you, will you be *happy*? You see, the seeds for being *happy* and the seeds for being *rich* are *different* seeds—and that explains why wealthy people can sometimes be so utterly unhappy.

The karmic seed that's planted by training ourselves to be satisfied with any level of material comfort is different. This seed ripens as pure *contentment*, and it's worth a huge amount of wealth seeds. A person who is contented with simplicity has surpassed wealth itself.

It really is true that there is no school like being put into difficult situations and learning to excel because of them. Karmically speaking, the decision to commit ourselves to something that is truly meaningful forces a lot of old, very dangerous seeds to go off—prematurely, but much more gently than they would have otherwise. It's sort of like the inconvenience of missing a flight that ends up crashing.

Finding Your Guardian Angel

II.44–45 If you engage in regular study,
then you come to be with
the Angel of your deepest dreams.
If you seek your Master's blessing,
you attain final meditation.

Svadhyayad ishtadevata samprayogah.
Samadhi siddhir ishvara pranidhanat.

The serious study of the spiritual classics—burning the midnight oil in the pleasant company of the greatest Masters of history—is not much in vogue in our times. Perhaps it's because knowledge has come to be associated with universities and degrees, rather than years of deeply fulfilling apprenticeship under a true Master.

At any rate, a real Master will demand from us—often painfully so—that we put our studies into actual practice. Which with yoga means an incessant examination of our inner weaknesses: a joy in exposing them and routing them out.

As we gradually replace our mental stockpile with an increasingly higher percentage of pure seeds, then our Master begins to come to us in ever higher ways. At a very specific point, she comes to us as the one perfect angel who will guide us personally to our final paradise together.

This is not some wishful fairy-tale thinking. It is the hard, cold, practical, inevitable result of devoting ourselves to the task of cleaning up the seeds within our own mind.

60 Body Yoga

II.46–47 The poses bring a feeling
of well-being that stays with you.
They do so through a balance
of effort and relaxation;
and through endless forms
of balanced meditation.

Sthira sukham asanam.
Prayatna shaithilya-ananta
samapattibhyam.

These lines are the original source for the physical yoga poses as we know them today. Originally these were mostly different types of meditation postures and a few additional exercises that would give you the strength and flexibility to sit in unmoving meditation for long periods of time.

Here really begins the idea of working on the heart and mind by working from the outside, on the body. By placing the parts of our body into very specific positions, we purposely affect the inner channels. This facilitates the flow of inner wind, or *prana*. And because our very thoughts ride upon this *prana* inside the channels, we bring greater kindness and knowledge to our mind, by using our body.

Meditation is defined as maintaining a balance that avoids mental lethargy and hyperactivity. It is a delicate process of correction and countercorrection, like the constant left-and-right of our hands upon a steering wheel.

Through practice, we learn to keep a straight line; then we relax our effort and ride, lest the correcting itself become a distraction. With regular practice, body and mind achieve well-bring that really lasts. Ultimately we attain a higher well-being, as the channels themselves transform into light.

61 The Lie of Choices

*II.48 And there will come a time
when differences
no longer harass you.*

Tato dvandva-anabhighatah.

How exactly does this transformation happen? As we'll see in the next chapter, there are three primary wind channels within the body. The middle channel runs down the center of the back, following the spine. On either side of it run two lesser channels.

Remember the Great Mistake: how we try to get the things we want in the wrong way, like a child hitting a bad man on a movie screen. This then plants negative seeds that ripen into our very troubled world.

When we see things in a wrong way, the inner winds inside the two side channels are active. This is because they are tied to mistaken thoughts about how our world works, and these thoughts run in the same two channels.

The incredible magic of yoga is that it actually attacks negative thoughts on a physical level, as the exercises release blockages of inner winds in the side channels.

These blockages cause us to see things in a polarized way: this and that, me and you, what I want versus what you want. When the blocks are freed, then getting what you want becomes getting what I want, and we are both freed.

62 The End of Breath

*II.49 The breath is controlled when,
as you remain there,
the passing of your breath
in and out simply stops.*

*Tasmin sati shvasa prashvasayor
gati vichedah pranayamah.*

If we are doing our yoga exercises correctly then, the side channels open up, *which actually causes us to think more clearly and kindly.* If you're not getting this effect with your yoga, then you're not doing it properly. At the bottom of everything are self-control and commitments, the seeds creating the yoga poses: Am I taking care of other people, every day?

In addition to physical exercises that reach down to open the channels, there is an entire science of breathing that touches the inner winds themselves, linked to our thoughts within the channels. Although our breath is not the inner wind, the two are intimately connected. Whatever happens with one resonates with the other, like guitar strings tuned to the same note.

And so in one direction, working from the outside in, we can remain in a meditation posture or yoga pose and master our breath, which then calms the inner winds: when you stand and hold a horse's reins, the rider atop it is stilled. From the inside out, we can quiet the thoughts and thus the winds: when the rider is calm, the horse is too.

A totally calm and properly focused mind brings negative thoughts to a standstill, at which point the outer breath simply stops.

How to Breathe

II.50 Keep a close watch
on the breath;
outside or inside,
paused or being exchanged.
Observe too
the place in the body,
the duration, and the count.
Long and fine.

Bahya-abhyantara stambha virttih
desha kala sankhyabhih
paridirshto dirgha sukshmah.

So the breath is connected to the inner winds, which are linked to our very thoughts. This means that if we keep a close eye on our breath—both during our yoga exercises and throughout the day as well—then we can monitor the state of our mind and the condition of those two troublesome side channels.

If you think about it, breath can be in three places: all breathed out, when it pauses momentarily; all breathed in—again a pause; or moving between these two states.

In meditation, in a yoga pose, and with the boss at work we strive to keep our breaths long and slow, with a constant even inflow and exhale. This keeps the inner winds calm and thus our mind clear and focused.

When we're nervous or upset, inhales tend to go much quicker than exhales. We correct this by mentally counting the seconds for each, until inhales and exhales take equal time. Then extend the calm exhales further.

Since the inner winds are tied to our thoughts, with proper training we can also mentally direct a certain number of breaths through specific inner blockages, and then the inner winds will follow.

Breathing to a Single Point

*II.51–53 The fourth state is where one has given up
outside, inside, and the experience itself.
And then one can destroy the veil that covers the light.
The mind is fit for focus.*

Bahya-abhyantara vishaya kshepi chaturthah.
Tatah kshiyate prakasha-avaranam.
Dharanasu cha yogyata manasah.

So the breath can be outside, inside, or experienced as moving between the two. But there's also that fourth possibility, when it stops
altogether.

We experience something close to this when we are reading a
really good book, or trying hard to hear a faint sound. The closer we
concentrate, the more calm the inner winds become, and thus the
breath. When the breath actually stops for long periods of time, it
does so for one of two reasons: either our focus in general is perfect,
or we have destroyed the very thoughts and winds that create the veil
of the Great Mistake.

Of course the first can help us get to the second, but it's the second one we want: that's what Master Patanjali defined as yoga itself,
back in the beginning. All the physical practices of yoga are aimed at
stilling the side channels, which causes us to see ultimate reality and
eventually turns our body into light: an angel who appears wherever
someone needs.

These results in physical yoga, and especially the breath exercises,
come only after steady work with a qualified teacher. Someone who's
been trained personally by a Master in an authentic tradition.
Someone who's obviously keeping up a good practice, and gotten results. Don't try to force things yourself, or do them incorrectly; you
could very well hurt your body or mind. Success comes very surely
and naturally only by planting the right seeds—through the yoga of
self-control and commitments.

65 Ending the Tyranny of Stimulation

II.54–55 Learn to withdraw the mind
from your physical senses;
freed from its ties to outer objects,
the mind can arrive
at its own real nature.
And with that, you attain
the highest control of the senses.

Svavishaya-asamprayoge chittasya
svarupa-anukara ivendriyanam
pratyahara.
Tatah parama vashyatendriyanam.

And so we have finished the first four of the five "outer" limbs of yoga: self-control, commitments, yoga exercises, and breathing practices. There's obviously a progression here; for example, the very act of being careful not to hurt others—purposefully planting good seeds—*is the only way* to get good at yoga exercises. But being sure to breathe calmly reaches back and *allows* you to be nice to others. And so each of the eight limbs supports each of the others, creating a self-perpetuating, upward spiral in our lives.

Here again, our physical senses are wonderful tools, and it's fine to enjoy a slice of pizza or a bowl of ice cream. To make serious progress in our goals of saving the universe, though, we have to manage these senses sensibly.

Enjoy a song fully and then turn off the radio, before it becomes background noise. Do your yoga exercises modestly but steadily, and you'll suddenly get cravings for the exact type of food, and the quantity of food, which is healthiest for you. Cultivate the art of happy silence, enjoyed with friends.

Eventually these will lead to the highest form of silence: direct communion with the ultimate.

Third Cornerstone

The Chapter on Practice

66 Focus and Stay

III. 1–2 Locking the mind
on an object is focus.
And staying on that object
over a stretch of time is fixation.

Tirtiyo Vibhuti Padah

Desha bandhash chittasya dharana.
Tatra pratyayaika dhyanam.

The third cornerstone for the house of yoga consists of the three inner limbs or practices, along with their practical applications. At the end of the last chapter we were learning to control our senses, which brings us automatically to focus. It's like finding your friend in a crowd at the train station.

On one level, the mind focuses on a single object through the process of eliminating all other objects around it: everything is the opposite of all that it's not. You check and eliminate faces in the crowd, and steadily narrow your focus down to your friend's face.

The more faces there are to weed out, the more difficult it is to find your friend. The more objects you possess in your house; the more unimportant things you have to do all day; the more useless news you've heard and the more you meet with others for unmeaningful talk, then the less chance you'll be able to focus.

Once we reach a single point, we need to stay there, threading that path between thinking of other things and dozing off mentally. Thinking of death fixes the first; thinking of destiny fixes the second.

67 The Clear Light

III.3 *Perfect meditation
then sees this same object
as its simple self:
its clear light,
totally void
of any nature of its own*

*Tad eva-artha matra
nirbhasam svarupa shunyam
iva samadhih.*

At some point, through a modest but very regular daily practice of meditation (performed according to the authentic instructions of that qualified teacher), we attain total stillness of the mind: focus that is fixed.

They say that stopping the Great Mistake is like chopping down a big tree. Perfect focus and the ability to stay are like two strong arms. But however strong we may be, we can't simply push a tree down. We need a very sharp ax.

To make meditation perfect, it's not enough to simply mentally stare at something like our breath for a long time. The mind even then is making its constant, deadly error, and we must fix it or come to the end of our life unfulfilled.

As we meditate we need to strive to see the one thing that is simply... missing, clear gone. We need to realize that nothing is anything; that is, even the hotness of a fire never *belonged* to it. It is *I* who make fire hot.

68 The Eye of Wisdom

III.4–8 When these three act together
as one, we call it "the combined effort."
When you master this skill,
you gain the eye of wisdom.
This is divided into various levels.
Relative to those that precede them,
these three are "inner" limbs.
But they are also "outer" limbs compared
to the state where the seeds are gone.

Trayam ekatra sanyamah. Taj jayat prajnya-alokah.
Tasya bhumishu viniyogah. Trayam antar angam
purvebhyah. Tad api bahir angam nirbijasya.

An ax lifted high with two strong arms has a certain undeniable power to it. You have ability to put your mind on a single point and to keep it there unwavering for an hour or more. At the same time, *you totally understand* where the thing you're focused on is really coming from—and not coming from. These three together—focus, fixation, and wisdom—represent a kind of teamwork or combined effort that will literally save your life, and the lives of many others.

Now you possess a truly powerful weapon, the one and only weapon that can destroy the pain of our world. This is the eye of wisdom—a metaphorical third eye—the light of knowledge within our deepest mind.

The three begin as an intellectual experience, and then a direct one, of ultimate reality. They combine with ultimate love and lead us through progressively higher levels of giving, ethical living, patience, effort, concentration, and understanding.

Compared to all that we have ever been—compared even to the first five practices of yoga—the combination of these three limbs is literally the most precious thing in the world. But even they are as the mind of a child compared to where they will take us.

69 The End of Thoughts?

III.9–10 The stopping occurs
according to whether the seeds for rising from it
or remaining within it are suppressed or manifest.
Its duration thus follows upon the mind.
This we call "the transformation of the stopping."
The termination, or elimination,
of negativities due to this
also depends upon the seeds.

Vyutthana nirodha sanskarayor
abhibhava pradurbhavau nirodha
kshana chitta-anvayo nirodha parinamah.
Tasya prashanta vahita sanskarat.

How does the team of perfect stillness and swordlike wisdom do its work? One day, after much practice and study—and if we've planted the necessary seeds by serving others—then we rise into an extraordinary meditation. Outside of time itself, we commune with ultimate reality, for the first time. After a brief while, we return.

There is a similar but infinitely less important experience where we fall into a deep, nearly unconscious state of meditation. We may awaken from this meditation hours later, and it feels like only a moment has passed: as if our mind itself had stopped.

But in neither meditation has the mind actually stopped. In the higher one, the Great Mistake has stopped for a while; in the lower one, only our surface consciousness has been suspended. In both cases we can only stay "in" as long as our seeds allow us: there is no conscious effort to awaken.

Stopping the Great Mistake completely, even for a few minutes the first time, eliminates certain negative thoughts forever. But again, their eternal absence also relies on seeds.

Using stillness and wisdom, to see thus how thoughts can pause, transforms the experience into the higher version.

70 How Things Begin and End

III.11–12 *What we call*
"the transformation of meditation"
is a single-pointedness toward all existing objects,
where the mind is also stopped, or resumes;
again according to these two.
And what we call "the transformation of single-pointedness"
is where that state of mind itself
either rests or arises, according again
to the same two factors.

Sarva-arthaika-agra tayoh kshayodayau
chittasya samadhi parinamah.
Tatah punah shantoditau tulya pratyayau
chittasyaika-agrata parinamah.

And so we may experience deep states of meditation where our mind seems to be stopped. It's important to use our higher stillness and meditation to understand the experience and transform it into something that can really help us with more serious issues, such as stopping pain and death itself.

The question then becomes how long we can stay in a place where the Great Mistake has stopped. The answer, for the first time, is that we stay only for a few minutes. Our pure seeds are still too fragile to maintain the stopping: they spend themselves; the stopping stops; and the Great Mistake resumes, despite ourselves.

During these few minutes, other powerful but fragile seeds have maintained both the meditational wisdom and the single-pointed stillness upon which it rests: our old team. They too though are at the mercy of their respective seeds—seeds to start, and seeds to stop.

We transform the pair as well then when we turn them upon themselves, realizing fully that realization can last only as long as our seeds do. This in turn sends us back to work on the first two limbs of yoga: planting seeds by taking care of others.

71 How Things Neither Begin Nor End

III.13–15 These are called "transformations"
because they create a change in the very condition
of the qualities of things,
whether external elements or internal powers.
All these things follow upon
a single thing they possess:
the fact that neither their stopping nor their starting
can ever be pointed to.
The cause for their other stages
follows too from the transformation.

Etenu bhutendriyeshu dharma
lakshana-avastha parinama vyakhyatah.
Shantodita-avyapadeshya dharma-anupati dharmi.
Krama-anyatvam parinama-anyatve hetuh.

It's crucial to realize that *the simple act of understanding a thing can transform its very condition.* People who truly *understand* external physical elements like water can, through that act of understanding, change the water into something solid and walk upon it. By *understanding* the sense power of vision, they can see around the world, or cure the blind.

All such transformations are possible only because all things are as they are at the mercy of one other thing. And this is the fact that no thing ever begins or ends. Nor does it pass through any other stage, like staying.

Focus your mind upon the exact moment you read this . . . word. But there was a part of this moment when you *started* to see the w, and a later part of the moment when you finished seeing the w.

And so on, infinitely. We can't be seeing what we're seeing, because there's no point where we *started* to see it. If we do see words—and we do—then it can be only because our mind has placed them down here upon the page.

The Power to Save
the World

III.16—18 The transformation of the combined effort
allows one to see both past and future.
At some point you are able to sort out the confusion,
where factors such as terms and objects
are mixed up, one with the other.
If you turn the combined effort on this, then you gain
the ability to know all the languages of livingkind.
Making it manifest as a present seed allows you to see past lives.

Parinama traya sanyamad atita-anagata jnyanam.
Shabda-artha pratyayanam itaretara-adhyasat sankara
tat pravibhaga sanyamat sarva bhuta ruta jnyanam.
Sanskara sakshat karanat purva jati jnyanam.

If things actually *begin* only due to a tiny mental picture we impose upon two otherwise unrelated microseconds, then what things *become* when they finish beginning has to come from the same place. When you truly understand this, you can turn bricks into gold.

But would you want to? With the unbearable emotional and physical pain that tears at every single person in this world, we would be compelled to use our abilities for a higher purpose. And so we begin the description of how we use the combination of stillness and wisdom to gain the powers of an angel.

If one moment in time is only a perception, then all moments are, and we could learn to see ahead and backward in time, to help people. We would also learn that we are mistaking our tiny mental pictures for "actual" objects. Since these pictures are what words are, we would then gain power over words themselves: the ability to speak to all people, guide all people, in their own language.

Transforming past and future seeds into present ones, we can describe to people the events of their past lives and our own, so they can grasp how everything comes from the way we've treated others.

73
Reading the Minds of Others

III.19–20 With the necessary cause,
one can read the minds of others.
This though is not done
through the one they're based in,
because of the fact that
it would then not be
their own experience.

Pratyayasya para chitta jnyanam.
Na cha tat sa-alambanam,
Tasya-avishaya bhutatvat.

In the previous chapters we spoke about the Path of Seeing: that brief period when we commune with ultimate reality. In the hours after this experience, we temporarily gain the ability to read other people's minds. As we progress through the next path, this ability becomes more and more stable.

Again, it's not that we can share mental seeds that are based or located in another person. Seeds in our own mind can be put there only by our own actions toward others. If this were not the case, then we simply wouldn't be here in this broken world. Masters of the past, in their infinite compassion, would have given us their own perfect seeds long ago.

And so reading another person's thoughts—and we really do—comes from our own seeds; if it came from theirs, then they wouldn't be having the thoughts.

Reading other people's minds—or even just sincerely trying to—is an important skill if we have something precious to teach them. We can peek in and see what they enjoy, and what they hope for, and the extent at that moment of their capacity to digest ideas.

74 The Power of Invisibility

III.21–22.a If one turns the combined effort
upon the body's visible form,
then one can attain invisibility,
since the eye becomes disassociated
from the object appearing to it,
as the power to grasp unto
this object is suspended.
The powers of shutting off
sound and the rest
are explained in the same way.

Kaya rupa sanyamat
tad grahya shakti stambhe chakshuh
prakasha-asamprayogentardharam.
Etena shabdadyantardhanam uktam.

People who are advanced in the path gain the power to become invisible whenever they wish to. Again, this is a matter of consciously manipulating how the pieces of an object—such as the color and outline of one's own body—are organized into that object by the mind. And this can be done only if the correct seeds have been planted. And this can be done only if one has been good to others: good enough to see them not see you, if that could help them.

We should say here that not everyone who possesses powers such as invisibility necessarily fully understands where they come from, how to keep them, or how to use them to help others. Sometimes a miracle may happen to us simply because of some old good seeds suddenly ripening—but if we don't understand the process, we can't repeat it.

People who meditate very regularly, even if they only use meditation to "space out" for a while, may temporarily gain a few powers. This is because, in any deep state of meditation, we simply cannot commit the negative actions and thoughts toward others that keep us from these powers.

Where It All Leads

*III.22.b When you turn the combined effort upon
those karmic seeds that will open
and those that will not,
then you gain the ability
to see their final outcome.
This can also be done
by the reading of omens.*

Sopakramam nirupakramam cha
karma tat sanyamad aparanta jnyanam.
Arishtebhyo va.

You buy your mother-in-law a new shower mat, in the hopes that she might like you more. The next day she slips on it and hurts herself.

We know enough by now, about how things really work, to know that she didn't slip because of the mat—but rather because of something negative she herself did to someone prior to that. And our good intentions *cannot* go wrong: the desire to please her will bring us many good things in the future.

Which doesn't change the fact that *it would be nice to know*, with confidence, the exact final consequences we can expect from any particular action we undertake. Someone who really understands how the seeds work can perceive which seeds in the storehouse will eventually open and sprout and which will forever lie unopened.

This is because *merely failing to understand* how the seeds work is *what* makes impure seeds viable and potent. Remove the Great Mistake, and old bad seeds never go off.

There are specific methods for using omens to see what might happen—such as foretelling death from people's shadows. In the end these too work only if we have the right seeds, from taking care of others.

The True Source of Power

III.23–25 The powers are to be found
in love and the rest.
And in these powers
lie the powers of the War-Elephant,
and all the others too.
If you place your eye on the true causes,
then you gain the ability to perceive
even very subtle things at a great distance away.

Maitryadishu balani.
Baleshu hasti bala-adini.
Pravirttyaloka nyasat sukshma
vyavahita viprakirshta jnyanam.

It's obvious by now that the extraordinary, unexpected powers we might want to seek in order to be of service to others all come from planting the right seeds. And so here the Master reminds us of the very most powerful way of planting these seeds: the practice of the Four Infinite Thoughts, from the first chapter.

Infinite love, which wants to give all living beings everything their heart desires. Infinite compassion, which wants to remove their tiniest little pain. Infinite joy, which wants to take them to a higher happiness than just houses and hamburgers: to a place of infinite happiness, beyond all fear or death. And infinite equanimity, which wants to do this for everyone, not just friends or family.

In Master Patanjali's day, an elephant was the ultimate war machine, powerful enough to destroy any obstacle. And so a being who had reached spiritual perfection was called a War-Elephant. When we transform into this angel, we will have ultimate powers: ultimate compassion; a knowledge of all things; and the ability to show ourselves anywhere in the universe, any time, to help others.

This is the true evolution of all the powers. You will see a child fall from worlds away, and be there to catch him or her, before you think to.

The Channel of the Sun

III.26 Turn the combined effort
upon the sun,
and you will understand
the earth.

Bhuvana jnyanam
surye sanyamat.

Back in the second chapter, when we spoke about the physical yoga exercises, we mentioned three main channels where inner wind, or *prana*, travels through the body. It's crucial to understand these channels, because we can then control our very thoughts, which are linked to the winds. We actually work on the physical body to stop the Great Mistake of the mind.

The central channel follows the spine; slightly to our right of it runs the sun channel. Tied to the winds that flow in this channel travel our "hot" negative thoughts: anger, hatred, jealousy, all based on disliking objects, events, and people because we fail to understand how we ourselves have produced them.

Stilling the turbulence of inner winds within the sun channel has the effect of freeing us from misunderstanding our outer reality: the world, the earth. The beauty of yoga is that we work on this channel simply and effectively through selected physical yoga exercises.

Breath control, practiced with authentic guidance, further achieves this goal. And then finally we use the teamwork of the last three limbs of yoga—mental focus, fixation, and wisdom—to still the sun channel from the inside.

78 The Channel of the Moon

*III.27 You will understand
the arrangement of the stars
if you turn this same effort
upon the moon.*

Chandre tara vyuha jnyanam.

To the left side of the central channel runs the channel of the moon. If the sun channel, which is bloodred, carries largely male energy—externally focused and action-oriented—then the milky-colored moon channel carries mostly female energy—introspective and thinking-oriented.

Within this channel run all our thoughts of liking things in the wrong way because we misunderstand them: taking the last maple-covered donut for ourselves.

When our yoga practice stills the winds in the moon channel, the very root of these thoughts is stopped. This is the tendency to see ourselves and our own mind—all the tiny sparks or stars of consciousness within us—as something too that comes from its own side, and not from our seeds.

Something to realize here: the very seeds that create us create our world. The seeds that create the first division of all—the channels of sun and moon within our very bodies—also make us male or female. They create day and night, sun and moon, you and me, earth and stars. The state of our world is a perfect reflection of the state of our channels, and thus our hearts.

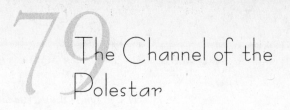

The Channel of the Polestar

*III.28 Turn the effort
upon the polestar,
and you will understand
their workings.*

Dhruve tad gati jnyanam.

The central channel, colored like crystal flame, runs up and down the body like the great axis around which the stars turn. It follows the line of the spine from between our legs to the tip of our head, curving down to a point between the eyebrows.

Linked to the winds in this channel run all our good thoughts: caring for others, watching what they want and need, and most important the realization that this in itself will literally create a perfect world.

The three channels are joined together below the area of our navel. Simply reading and understanding the words on this page sucks inner wind, or *prana*, out of the troublesome side channels and directs it into the pure central channel. This in turn further reveals to us the workings of earth and stars.

You must realize that the true purpose of all physical yoga practice is to guide inner wind out of the side channels and into the central channel. This triggers our progress through all five paths, especially the direct perception of ultimate reality.

When *all* the inner wind dissolves into the central channel, the body changes from flesh to light, and you stand upon all worlds.

80 Choke Points and Chakras

III.29–31 Turn the same effort
upon the wheel at the navel,
and you will understand
the structure of the body.
Turn it upon the throat,
and you put an end
to hunger and thirst.
This is a stable state
of the channels of the turtle.

Nabhi chakre kaya vyuha jnyanam.
Kantha kupe kshut pipasa nivirttih.
Kurma nadyam sthairyam.

As they follow the central channel up the body, the two side channels twist around it at certain spots, like vines. This creates choke points that obstruct the flow of winds within the central channel, thus hindering the sweet and wise thoughts linked to these winds.

During the development of the inner channels within the fetus, pressure builds up at these choke points, and secondary channels spurt out from them. Looking down the spine, these are seen radiating out like the spokes of a wheel. Thus they are called *chakras*, from the Sanskrit word for "wheel."

The first wheel to form in the womb is at the navel. Eventually an entire network develops, and the very structure of our skeleton, blood vessels, and nervous system forms around the channels, like ice around the contours of a twig. This means that any physical ailment we ever have can be traced to the channels, and cured, with understanding.

Turning this understanding upon the *chakra* at the neck allows us, in time, to overcome even the need to eat. We gradually control all five physical senses, which are tied to five secondary winds such as the "turtle" wind, responsible for hearing and related to our turtle-shaped liver.

8 Everything from Understanding

III.32–34 *Turn it upon the radiance*
at the tip of the head,
and you will see the powers.
All of them come
from total understanding.
Turn it upon the heart,
and you will know the mind.

Murdha jyotishi siddha darshanam.
Pratibhad va sarvam.
Hirdaye chitta sanvit.

The inner wheels, or *chakras,* begin as choke points, but the very act of focusing upon them with understanding releases the tightness of the two side channels wrapped around them.

Think of the inner wind, or *prana,* within the three main channels as being a certain fixed amount, like the air inside a toy animal made of long thin balloons. If you squeeze the tummy, the legs get fatter.

If you work on a choke point with thoughts of knowledge and caring for others, inner wind leaves the side channels that caused the choke point in the first place. The *chakra* then becomes a center of radiance and high spiritual realizations.

Using this method, we can release a radiant, white, honeylike substance within the *chakra* at the tip of our head. This triggers worldly powers, and then divine ones. Again, all the powers ultimately support and also spring from a clear understanding of the seeds as they create the world.

Within the *chakra* at the heart lies an indestructible drop of consciousness, infinitely smaller than the tip of a needle. Herein lies the storehouse of billions of seeds, projecting forth our life. When this *chakra* heart is opened, ultimate love bursts forth as crystal light.

Know Thyself

III.35 The causes for reality and the person,
however very distinct from one another
these two may be, are no different.
We experience them not because
of something outside of ourselves,
but as something from ourselves.
Turn the combined effort upon this,
and you will understand the person.

Sattva purushayor atyanta-asankirnayoh
pratyaya-avishesho bhogah
para-arthatvat sva-artha sanyamat
purusha jnyanam.

It's a lot easier to deal with the misunderstanding of our outer reality, which runs in the sun channel, than to correct the misunderstanding of the person—meaning ourselves—which runs in the moon channel.

Take the outer reality of a pen, for example. If I hold a pen up to you and ask you what it is, you automatically say "A pen." And in that split second you also believe that it's a pen from its own side. You think that "pen-ness" is somehow coming out of the pen itself.

But if we hold the same object up to a dog, he simply sees it as a mildly interesting stick: perhaps something good to chew on.

A moment's reflection tells us that neither view of the object is more "correct." And we also quickly see that "pen-ness" is not exuding from the pen. Rather, "pen" is a perfect little idea-picture imposed upon a shiny cylinder by my own mind. And *which* picture my mind comes up with all depends on the seeds—on how I've treated others.

That's in fact what *makes* me a human, and the dog a dog. Even the question of whether you can *think* these ideas is coming from the seeds.

When Two Is One

III.36–37 With this you develop
supernormal abilities of hearing,
touch, sight, taste, and smell.
During meditation,
these could be an obstacle;
when you rise from meditation,
they are powers.

Tatah pratibha shravana
vedana-adarsha svada
varta jayante.
Te samadhau upasarga
vyutthane siddhayah.

The ability to understand a simple pen then is a powerful tool that allows us to go behind reality and make adjustments at its very core: sort of like having the source code for a computer program, or working on an organism at the level of its genetic code.

The distances at which we can hear two other people having a conversation is an example. If a certain number of feet were inherently the number of feet at which we can no longer hear what they're saying, then someone standing next to us who has much more acute hearing than us shouldn't be able to hear them either. Just like the pen and the dog.

And so rather than bringing about some miraculous change in our ability to hear, we simply replace the seeds in our own mind that are creating the *limit* at which we can hear. A hundred feet becomes two feet, and we can listen to people talking two houses down the street.

This could obviously drive you mad, and make activities like sleep and meditation impossible. Generally speaking, we are automatically protected by the fact that such powers are only gained through the desire to use them to serve others.

The Rainbow in a Prison

III.38 When you loosen the ties
that bind you,
and know this for a prison,
then you can send your mind
to enter another body.

Bandha karana shaithilyat
prachara sanvedanach cha
chittasya parasharir aveshah.

We dearly love our bodies of flesh and blood, but imagine how they would seem to a person whose body had already changed to light. Sort of a slimy prison. A dangerous place to be stuck in.

Incidentally, you maintain the general outer form of a human being when your body does change. Other people (remember the pen and the dog) might even see you the same as before. You and others like you, though, see you as the most exquisite being you can imagine right now, magnified a thousand times over.

And so sometimes the body of light is called the "rainbow" body, because from a distance a rainbow looks like solid stuff, but up close you can pass your hand through it: no more guts and blood.

Since a dog in the end is only the seeds to see things as a dog, a person again who really understands seeds could take on various outer forms, and appear to be born as various different people, if this would help us. He knows it's easier for us, on a day-to-day level, to relate to someone fairly much like ourselves. And so at the beginning he comes to us that way.

The Five Primary Winds

*III.39–40 When you gain mastery
over the upward-running wind,
then you can pass unimpeded over
bodies of water, swamps,
thornbushes, and the like.
When you gain mastery
over the co-resident wind,
you gain inner fire.*

*Udana jayaj jala pangka
kantaka-adishvasanga utkrantish cha.
Samana jayat prajvalanam.*

When the inner winds race to a specific part of the body and gather there, even momentarily, to perform a necessary bodily function, we identify them as one of the five primary winds.

The first of these, the "pervasive" wind, covers the entire body, governing the flow of all other winds to whatever place they are needed. The "life" wind maintains life itself and also the passage of breath. The "downward-clearing" wind ensures the elimination of feces and urine.

The "upward-running" wind mentioned here relates to eating and speaking, also assisting the upward movement of any other wind. When with knowledge of seeds we gain mastery over this wind, we can move quickly—even over obstacles like lakes or thick brush—if someone needs help. In our final evolution, we pass through planets and galaxies at the speed of thought—the speed of a seed ripening.

The final primary wind "resides together" with both digestive fire and mystic fire near the navel. On the first level, it distills nutrients from food and distributes them throughout the body. On the second level, it triggers a downward flow of the radiant nectar from the tip of the head, engendering knowledge, bliss, and our angelic transformation.

86 The Three Skies

*III.41–42 When you turn the combined effort
upon the relationship between
the ear and space, you gain
the angel power of hearing.
When you turn this effort
upon the relationship between
the body and space, you gain
a power of meditation where you become
light as a wisp of cotton,
and can thus fly through the sky.*

*Shrotra-akashayoh sambandha
sanyamad divyam shrotram.
Kaya-akashayoh sambandha sayamal
laghu tula samapattesh cha-akasha gamanam.*

The word here for "space" had three meaning in ancient times. One was simply sky, space, the distance between things.

The second meaning, as we've mentioned before, was place itself: that unchanging thing which objects enter, stay in, and then exit.

The third was space in the sense of the void that's left when you find out that something you thought was there never was. The feeling you get when you reach into your pocket after a meal at an expensive restaurant and realize you've left your wallet at home.

We get the same feeling of absence when we realize that everything around us is not coming *at* us, but *from* us. Seeing how this space allows us to hear, seeing how this space allows our body to be there, allows us again to adjust the "switches" on both these objects. Unheard switched to heard, heavy switched to light.

Again we use the resulting powers first to help a limited number of people. As we grow, the number becomes infinite. All the powers evolve this way—from mundane, to helpful, to enlightened. In the end the mind flies free through the sky of what was never there anyway.

The Four Bodies

*III.43–44 Those who no longer perceive
anything as being outside
experience the transformation
into the ultimate body.
With this, every veil that covers the light
is destroyed.
Turn the combined effort
upon the fact that this gross body is an object
that comes from that subtle nature,
and you'll gain mastery over the elements.*

*Bahir akalpita virtti mahavideha
tatah prakasha-avarana kshayah.
Sthula svarupa
sukshma-anvaya-arthavattva
sanyamad bhuta jayah.*

These lines mark the point at which the combined effort of stillness and understanding has been sustained for so long that we undergo the final transformation, into a being who can serve all worlds. At this point we will have four distinct parts, or bodies.

In a way, we already possess the first part of an angel, and we always have. It is *the simple fact that we are not what we are:* you are not the person they give that word, your name. Rather, the name—the seed picture—came first, and then made you you. Since you are not you any other way, you are available to become something else—an angel. And you always have been. This is your first body.

When we grasp that the way we *look*—our physical appearance—is also available in the same way, we begin the hard work of collecting enough seeds to change the actual physical elements of our body into those of the angel.

88 The Last One Left

III.45–46 With this you attain
power at microscopic levels
and all the rest.
You achieve a perfect body,
which cannot be hurt
by any existing thing.
You gain the body of perfection:
exquisite in its appearance,
strong, solid as diamond itself.

Tatonima-adi pradurbhavah kaya sampat
tad dharma-anabhighatash cha.
Rupa lavanya bala
vajra sanhananatvani
kaya sampat.

There is a traditional list of eight low-level powers that we can use to help others in a limited way: the ability to shrink and pass through a crack, or to lighten your body and fly through the air—the types of powers mentioned earlier.

By this stage though we have reached the ultimate evolution of these powers, which is the second body of the angel: billions of different physical forms that we send out. Imagine the ability to appear as a pet dog to a lonely person, or even as their favorite television show.

Then imagine filling an entire world with different beings, all interacting with each other; plus all the things they use every day. For a finished yogi, the first is considered "small" stuff; the second is "lightweight."

And so I really could be the last person left here who hasn't turned into an angel.

At the center of all these forms that the angel is sending out sits the "home" body. This is the third body, the paradise body, exquisite and indestructible. And she will never leave us, until we become her.

The Body of All-Knowing

III.47–48 If you turn the combined effort
upon the fact that the senses
which hold onto objects also follow
upon their true nature, their real self,
then you gain mastery over the powers of sense.
Thus then you also master
that thing which takes
the aspect: the main thing,
the swift messenger of the mind.

Grahana svarupa-asmita-anvaya-arthavattva
sanyamad indriya jayah.
Tato mano javitva vikarana bhavah
pradhana jayash cha.

So far we have attained three bodies: the "emptiness" body, which makes all the other ones possible, plus two physical bodies: one that we send out in infinite forms; and another that we stay in ourselves, within our heaven.

The fourth body then is the body of what our mind will become. Our sense powers take hold of objects and then report back to the mind. The mind, as we'll see more fully in the last chapter, is like a mirror, assuming the form or aspect of whatever the senses present to it. When you see a red apple, a part of your mind is in a sense imbued with redness.

It takes a split second for the mind to identify the objects presented to it—including organizing thought-sounds into thought-words. So in one way we're always a split second behind what's going on around us, but the principal character, mind, is so quick that we never notice.

In the last chapter we'll see how the true nature of every part of this process is that it's still coming *from* the mind. Understanding this allows us to reach the fourth body: the power to know all things.

Herein Lies Total Purity

III.49–50 *This then becomes the support*
of all things, and a knower
of all things; for all things—
whether the reality around us
or the people themselves—
are nothing more than its manifestations.
And if we can avoid attachment even to this,
we can destroy all the negative seeds.
Herein lies total purity.

Sattva purusha-anyata-akhyati
matrasya sarva bhava-adhishthatirtvam
sarvajnyatirtvam cha.
Tad vairagyad api dosha bija
kshaye kaivalyam.

The Master again summarizes the only way that we could reach the four bodies of an angel. In the end, the mind underlies all things—projecting everything we are aware of, even ourselves. At the end, the mind then fulfills its true capacity, of seeing directly every one of these objects—past, present, or future.

In one final mental twist, we need to understand that even our *understanding* of how all this works is *itself* a projection: a mental picture presented to our mind when extraordinarily rare and powerful seeds break open.

The ideas presented in Master Patanjali's little book on yoga, especially the description of the powers that we've just covered, are *coming from you.* Whether you grasp these ideas to fulfill the destiny of this world, or whether it all seems a little far-fetched this afternoon, is *also coming from you.*

Understanding this emptiness of understanding itself has the effect of destroying billions of old negative seeds within our mind. This in itself takes us a long way toward the final goal: total purity.

91 Respecting Our Destiny

III.51 And there will come a time
when they invite you
to take your place with them.
You must become a source
of pride for your family,
or you'll again fall victim
to all you sought to avoid.

Sthanyupanimantrane sanga
smaya-akaranam punah
anishta prasangat.

The minute you first picked up this book, you attracted the attention of some very important people: everyone who has studied the book in the last two thousand years, and understood it, and practiced it, and become the angel.

Simply by *thinking* the ideas we've read about so far, you have become part of a certain family of people. People who are very concerned about the pain of the world. People who have the spark of high understanding somewhere within them. Who believe that, somehow, there must be a *key* to stopping death and unhappiness altogether.

We said that we had to understand understanding itself; that it too is coming from seeds. And the only seeds it can come from are planted by wanting to be the one who rescues all the rest of us.

As your powers grow, and you evolve, your own physical and emotional pain will of course begin to disappear. There's a point at which you may get trapped, thinking to stop at that.

But then, you see, these important people will show themselves to you, and invite you into the higher family, which acts only for the happiness of the entire family—of livingkind.

The Final Moments

III.52–53 If you turn the combined effort
upon the two stages of this moment,
then you gain the knowledge
that comes from not discriminating.
You then attain the ability to be in the two equally,
unrestricted by anything: by birth, or type, or place.

Kshana tat kramayoh sanyamad
avivekajam jnyanam.
Jati lakskana deshair
anyata-anavachedat tulyayos
tatah pratipattih.

There are three crucial moments at the end, when we gain all four bodies.

The first is the last moment in which we are still not the angel: we are in what is called "the wisdom of the final instant." To get here we have seen the ultimate directly, on the Path of Seeing, briefly. And then we have worked our way up through seven levels, using what we saw, and discriminating—in the sense of staying aware that even now the way things look to us is not the way they really are.

During three more levels we need no longer discriminate this way: we no longer have the seeds for things to even *appear* to us in the wrong way. This brings us to that final moment; we cross over; and in the next moment we have this new knowledge—the power to know all things—born from the last three levels.

For one split second, we sit in but one exquisite body, in paradise. And then, because of the prayer we have made for countless lifetimes—to serve others—we without a single thought appear on all worlds, angelic.

93 All Things in All Ways

III.54–55 You attain the knowledge
that comes from discriminating;
the one that frees you,
where we are able to see all things
and the way all things are,
without having to alternate
between the two.
When the person
and the reality around that person
are equally pure,
this is total purity.

Tarakam sarva vishayam sarvatha vishayam
akramam cheti vivekajam jnyanam.
Sattva purushayoh shuddhi samye kaivalyam.

Before we reach the final goal, it is completely impossible to be in an experience of ultimate reality and still be experiencing the normal, deceptive reality around us now. And for us to experience ultimate reality, we must be in a state of deep meditation. And so we cannot help anyone if we are not practicing how to meditate ourselves, every day.

In a sense all things come from this basic ability to discriminate between the way we always thought things were happening and the way we realize they are really happening.

Even at very high levels then we can only alternate between seeing ultimate reality during deep meditation and being in deceptive reality at other times. This changes when we reach the body of the angel: then, and only then, we can see all things, and all creatures in the world, and love them completely, serve them, and in the same moment see their higher reality, absolute emptiness.

This very knowledge and love plants pure seeds that sustain it into the next moment, at which time its very existence again plants the seeds for it to be there in the following moment, on through eternity, total purity.

Fourth Cornerstone

The Chapter on Total Purity

94 We Must Become as Gardeners

*IV. 1–3 Powers can be attained either at birth, through herbs,
spells, extreme practices, or through deep meditation.
The transformation that occurs between births
is fulfilled by nature. In order to be released from them,
we must destroy the veil of the qualities of things.
And then we must become as gardeners.*

Chaturthah Kaivailya Padah

*Janmaushadhi mantra tapah samadhija siddhayah.
Jatyantara parinamah prakirtyapurat.
Nimittam aprayojakam prakirtinam
varana bhedas tu tatah kshetrikavat.*

The first chapter took us down the five paths, to perfection. The next
two chapters took us there through the eight limbs. The final chapter now takes us through the mental details to the same place.

There are many ways to the special powers we mentioned. If a
person is very attached to his house, for example, then after he dies
he may return as a spirit or ghost chained to the house, with powers
like walking through walls.

Deceased people in the spirit world, waiting for their next life, automatically gain similar powers, and try to contact loved ones. This
existence and its powers also end, by nature, within seven weeks.

One can moreover gain special powers and visions using herbs or
drugs, or through extreme practices like sleep deprivation or drastic
fasting. Or one can utter special spells to fly or pick up fire.

The problem with all these methods is that they simply cannot
be sustained at will. We must instead master deep meditation, and
see that the qualities which all things possess actually come from our
seeds. Then we must quietly, happily, and steadily tend the garden of
our own minds, to produce paradise.

The Destruction of the Storehouse

IV.4–6 Emanations are only possible
because of the self-nature
of the states of mind.
When you destroy
the mistaken attitude,
then the mind is released
from ideas of one or many.
Herein lies the destruction of the storehouse
attained through high meditation.

Nirmana chittanyasmita matrat.
Pravirtti bhede prayojakam
chittam ekam anekesham.
Tatra dhyanajam anashayam.

The one most important power from the last chapter was the ability to emanate, or send ourselves out to help one person, and later on infinite people. Each requires a certain state of mind called the "emanation state." We can only enter this state because its nature too is that it is produced by our kindness toward others.

A popular exercise in ancient times for seeing that things actually come from us was called "neither one nor many." You can't see a car without looking at its parts. But you can have all of the parts of a car and still not have a car—so the parts are not the car.

So if the parts you need to see aren't the car, then where is the car itself coming from? Needless to say, two or three such cars.

Grasp this about your mind itself—grasp this about the *idea* to send out countless clones of yourself to help people—and you are halfway there.

Meditating upon how things really work functions to destroy the storehouse of negative seeds, as we saw at the end of the first chapter. Gardening is both planting flowers and stopping weeds.

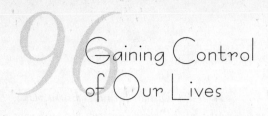

Gaining Control of Our Lives

IV.7–8 Deeds done by a true practitioner
are neither white nor black.
Those done by others are of three different kinds.
At that point, the corresponding consequences
that will ripen from these
are perfectly obvious to them
from the seeds they've planted.

Karma-ashukla-akirshnam yoginah
trividham itaresham.
Tatas tad vipaka-anugunanam
eva-abhivyaktir vasananam.

If our lives are actually run by old seeds sprouting in our mind, then logically life would be a little frustrating. Many of the immediate actions that we take then to get what we want simply wouldn't work out. And isn't that just the way it is?

Gardening your reality means taking back control over your life. It means knowing exactly how to get the things you want, because you now understand precisely what seeds to plant and how they will ripen. *This* is yoga; *this* is true practice.

Most people are constantly and blindly planting three kinds of seeds in their mental garden: many moment-to-moment little black negative seeds; a lot of "neutral" seeds that are planted by our constant, fundamental misunderstanding of things; and the occasional nice white seeds, from helping someone.

You must understand that even white seeds planted without *understanding* cause pain, because they wear out. Millions of white seeds have created your life, and it is leaking away as you read these words. True practitioners do the same good deeds with *understanding*; instead of planting impure white or black seeds, they plant only pure white ones, and thus run their lives themselves.

The End of Limits

IV.9–11 Distant lifetimes, distant places,
and distant times all become entirely here and now,
for the thought of them and the seeds for them
assume the exact same form.
They see them forever, back to no beginning,
ahead with nothing left.
The structure of causes and effects is maintained
by certain factors; it disappears then, when they do.

Jati desha kala vyavahitanam apyanantaryam
smirti sanskarayoh ekarupatvat.
Tasam anaditvam chashisho nityatvat.
Hetu phala-ashraya-alambanaih
sangirhitatvad esham abhave tad abhava.

You can recollect or think about your fantastic vacation spot right now, but it's not the same as being there—it's only a mental picture of being there. So if everything is just mental pictures anyway, why *isn't* it the same as being there?

When we *think* about a nice place, a seed has ripened in our mind to *imagine* it. When we are *sitting* in a nice place, a seed has sprouted to *be* there. And so (as you may have noticed) it doesn't matter how much you *want* to be there, you're not going to get there just by *wanting* to be.

The *only* way to get there is to purposefully plant the right seeds—say by providing a nice vacation for someone else. Then sit back and wait for the fireworks.

A person who's gotten very good at mental gardening though utilizes a powerful inner catalyst of knowledge and wanting to help others. She can then frame even distant events mentally, and thereby be there. She reaches backward and ahead into infinite time with nothing left unknown.

When misunderstanding stops, the old storehouse collapses, replaced by self-perpetuating, pure seeds.

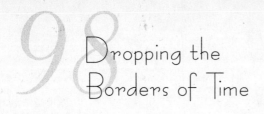

Dropping the Borders of Time

IV.12–14 It comes because those who understand things have broken through the idea that past and future are times that could exist in and of themselves. For them, the most subtle details of the very nature of things are evident. Since all the possible permutations of things are but one, their basis is suchness.

Atita-anagatam svarupatostyadhva bhedad dhar-manam. Te vyakta sukshma guna-atmanah. Parinamaikatvad vastu tattvam.

Here's another easy demonstration of emptiness. The boss bursts into your office and yells at you for blowing a customer's order.

In reality his face is only some reddish color, and his voice a certain number of decibels. But the seeds in your mind go off and impose upon this the finished image of an unpleasant person.

Someone else in the room may feel that he's being quite reasonable. That person's seeds are laying a different picture on him. Neither image is necessarily correct. It's not that unpleasantness or pleasantness is flowing from the boss. And that's his emptiness.

Ancient meditators were able to establish that the impression of time passing only occurs because of sixty-five separate images that go off in our mind every fingersnap; interestingly, about the number of frames per second in a film.

Time itself is just like the boss. How fast we see it pass—at the dentist or with a good friend—depends only upon our seeds. Those who see these subtle details can define their own time, by gardening.

Because emptiness is the foundation underlying all events, we are all capable of seeing everything that happens, in this one moment.

Beyond but Not Beyond the Mind

IV.15–16 Since the two states of mind
are distinct from one another,
they take separate routes
to experience this one same basis.
And it's not the case that any one state of mind
could, by way of something else,
experience this basis without a correct perception.
If that could happen, anything could happen.

Vastu samye chitta bhedat
tayor vibhakta panthah.
Na chaika chitta tantram vastu
tad apramanakam tada kim syat.

If emptiness is the most important thing—the foundation allowing all other things to happen—why is it so difficult for us to grasp?

For the answer, we return to the Great Mistake. We've said all along that—on one level—every single perception we ever have is mistaken. But if our mind is making some fundamental error every moment of our lives, then how can we ever *catch ourselves* making this mistake? The very instrument we're using is itself defective.

Some people claim that we never can see the truth with this defective mind. Others say we can, if we work by way of our self-awareness: a little independent corner of our mind that listens to and watches it, even though the mind itself never sees anything correctly.

The great Masters of history say that both of these ideas are silly. As Master Patanjali himself mentioned in the opening verses, there are two other routes for approaching the foundation truth of emptiness. One is reasoning—like an actor in a movie who explains to the audience how the movie can't be real. This leads to a direct, correct experience of ultimate reality during meditation, triggered by the purest of seeds.

How We Hear Ourselves Think

> IV.17–18 Whether the mind is aware
> of a basis—an object—or not depends upon
> its exposure to that object.
> The workings of the mind are always something
> that both are aware of,
> for this is not something
> that depends upon the degree
> to which each person has transformed herself.

Tad uparaga-apekshatvat
chittasya vastu jnyata-ajnyatam.
Sada jnyatash chitta
virttayas tat prabhoh
purushasya-aparinamitvat.

If you think about it a moment, it's clear that the only way we can say something exists is if we, or someone, know it. Perhaps not always directly, but at least through its effects: we "see" the wind blowing through the trees.

If there is a higher reality that saves us and underlies all things, then it must also support a perception of it. Objects depend upon subjects, and subjects rest upon objects. Neither can exist without the other. It's not true we can never see the truth.

The mind is like a mirror: place an object in front of it, and the mirror assumes the likeness of that object. It's not true that we can't watch our own mind simply with our own mind—even without some exotic bystander—to discover how it's making the Great Mistake. Everyone, regardless of her spiritual level, is watching her mind work all the time, including those on both routes to truth.

Our physical senses detect outer stimuli; our mental sense detects inner images and thoughts. In a millisecond, these as a group are presented to the mirror of our mind—and we see the world and ourselves.

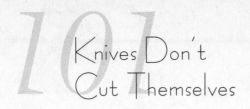

Knives Don't Cut Themselves

IV.19–20 This does not occur
because the mind is aware
of itself, since it would
then rather be
the object it was seeing.
And then, since they are
one and the same,
neither would be
what was holding the object.

Na tat svabhasam dirshyatvat.
Ekasamaye chobhaya-anavadharanam.

Subjects and objects then are necessarily different, and separate. The ancient Masters said that the mind is like a knife: it cannot cut itself. If the mind could see itself in a single moment, it couldn't be what was being seen, or what saw it.

Now, this doesn't at all contradict what we said back in the second chapter about the perception of separate subjects and objects being what causes all our problems. But here "separate" refers only to subjects and objects that aren't coming from the same place: from the seeds within our own minds.

It's important to realize that it's not at all the case that we are just living in our own minds, confined there forever. Outer objects and other people may be a result of images that I am creating, but that doesn't mean they're not real, that they don't exist "out there."

The seeds create them *as* out there. If you don't think so, go out and stand in front of a moving car. Its steel bumper, which your seeds are projecting, will strike your leg—which you are also projecting—and you'll go to a projected hospital and get a very *real* projected hospital bill.

The Apparent Self-Awareness

IV.21–22 When one is aware of things
within the mind itself, it must however be
both that which knows and that which is known;
this though is due to recollection and seeds.
The way in which the mind is aware of itself
is that it falls into believing the appearance that things
are arriving to it which it never sent out.

Chitta-antara dirshye buddhi buddher
atiprasangah smirti sanskarash cha.
Chiter apratisankrama-ayas
tad akara pattau
svabuddhi sanvedanam.

But if the mind can't see itself, how then can I be aware of myself at all? How can I listen to myself think?

Take a moment to think about how you hear yourself think. Listen to the thoughts in your mind.

Now—a question. Are you the one who is *saying* what you hear? Or are you the one *listening* to what you hear? You see the problem.

We are indeed though undeniably hearing ourselves think. What's actually happening is that seeds *from how we have treated others* are going off in our mind and presenting thoughts to the mirror of our mind. We are not thinking our thoughts—the seeds are.

But if that's the case, am I forever to be simply a helpless witness of what the seeds present to me—whether it's the outside world or my own thoughts? What happened to free will?

Come on, that's what this whole book has been about. You *can't* control the present moment. It's happening *to* you. It's like dry cement.

But you have every power and right—and you must *use* this power and right—to select what new seeds you plant in the garden of your mind.

How We Project the World

IV.23–24 The mind perceives
all of its objects
through the exposure
of what is seen
to what sees.
Countless seeds within our minds
make us see
the great variety of things around us.
The way it works
is that they organize
other parts in a certain way.

Drashtir dirshyoparaktam chittam sarva-artham.
Tad asankhyeya vasanabish chitram api
para-artham sanhatya karitvat.

We've established then that the mind sees everything it sees—even it-self—only when objects are presented to it, the subject.

Here the Master reminds us of where all these objects—and of course even the mirror itself—are coming from: countless seeds within our minds, planted there by how we have treated others. And so if you think about it, it makes perfect sense that real yoga doesn't begin with the third limb of yoga—the yoga exercises. Rather, it begins where it must: with the first limb, self-control, taking care of others.

You see, it's not that the physical yoga can do anything for you. It can't. It's empty: it could break your neck as easily as reduce your waistline. Whether yoga *works* on you—whether medicine works for you, whether your car starts today, whether the sun itself comes up tomorrow—all depends upon how the seeds organize your reality.

Nothing does anything to anything else. Nothing has any power to do anything. If anything works at all, it is only because we have cared for others.

Learning from Seeing

IV.25–26 *Those who have experienced*
the extraordinary vision
never stop meditating upon
the way the self really is.
Engrossed then in discrimination,
the mind is carried on
toward total purity.

Vishesha darshina atma bhava
bhavana vinivirttih.
Tada viveka nimnam
kaivalya pragbharam chittam.

In Master Patanjali's time, people didn't relate to books the way we do: to read once from cover to cover, put away, or toss out. A relationship with a really meaningful book was like a marriage. You sat down and read it, studied it—probably memorized most or all of it. You kept it with you, as a friend and help-mate, your entire life.

Now that you've read this book, you need to *use* it. You need to get through the five paths that every seeker must travel.

First you probably need a personal disaster—a divorce, or personal illness, or loss of a loved one—to get you asking questions, to pick the book up.

Second you need to study it carefully; seek out "live" guidance if you can. Spend a lot of time thinking about the seeds, and especially that idea of emptiness. You'll need to plant *new* seeds to grasp all this. Be *good* to people, dedicate it to understanding.

Third part: learn to meditate properly, work toward gaining ultimate love and seeing ultimate truth. About twenty minutes in this gets you to the fourth path, discriminating now between how things seem and how you know them to be different.

The End of Seeds

IV.27–28 Due to the seeds,
certain factors intervene
during intervals of that.
These are destroyed
in the same way described
for the negative thoughts.

Tach chidreshu pratyaya-antarani sanskarebhyah.
Hanam esham kleshavad uktam.

If the third path happens in minutes, traveling the entire length of the fourth path may take you a lifetime or more.

This is a period when, by tradition, the physical practices of yoga are very important: working from the outside in, as well as the inside out. Banging on the outside of a blocked pipe to clear it, as you push a stick down the inside at the same time. Working to loosen the choke hold of the side channels, the misunderstanding of subjects and objects: ourselves and our world.

At this point we possess the tools for working on the storehouse, but our work is still imperfect. The work itself can trigger minor explosions in the interim, like clearing an old minefield. We encounter obstacles, but we have seen how the end will be, and there is no despair.

Say you meet an angry person. How much longer can you get upset, knowing first that you have created him; and second that your old, natural reaction is precisely the one that will keep him in your world?

So first the negative emotions go, and then gradually all the seeds related to them—all killed by sheer understanding.

Debts Never Paid

*IV.29–30 You will never have to pay
those old debts back;
not a single one.
You have reached the meditation
of the galaxy of teachings,
a revelation into
the way of all things,
beyond all discrimination.
With this you destroy
all negative thoughts
and all ignorant deeds.*

*Prasankhyanepyakusidasya
sarvatha-aviveka khyater
dharma meghah samadhih.
Tatah klesha karma nivirttih.*

We spoke before about ten high levels of spiritual development. We reach the first one when we first see ultimate reality on the third path. Up through the seventh level, we are on the fourth path using what we understood about ultimate reality, keeping our mind on the distinction between what *seems* real and what *is* real.

Toward the end of the fourth path we pass through those three final levels—the "pure" levels—and destroy the last subtle seeds that limit us: everything at all related to old negative thoughts and actions. Whatever we have ever done wrong, in countless lifetimes, is forever cancelled and erased.

The tenth and final level—the very end of the fourth path—is called the "galaxy of the teachings." We are already capable of visiting the perfect paradises of angels who have come before us, to learn from them. We are on the threshold of releasing billions of copies of ourself into the universe, to share the teachings of this small book in showers of wisdom that spread like galaxies.

Stepping Over a Puddle

IV.31–32 And then you are freed
from the veil of impurity
that covers all things.
When knowledge is limitless
then all there is to know
is reduced to the size of a puddle.
At this point, those who have finished
what they set out to do accomplish
the perfection of qualities, which comes
from the stages of transformation.

Tada sarva-avarana mala-apetasya
jnyanasya-anantyaj jnyeyam alpam.
Tatah kirta-arthanam parinama
krama parisamaptir gunanam.

As a culture, we tend to think that we know more than people did before us because—well—we know *more* things. But there is also knowing a thing *well*: knowing how it really works. If we know this one thing, then knowing all the things there are to know, across the breadth of the ocean of this entire universe, becomes no more than stepping over a puddle of water.

Please don't be fooled by life, and by the small-minded people of the world, by skeptics, into believing that you are not capable of this, of becoming an actual angel, who sees all things and helps all living creatures.

This little book on yoga has lasted for two thousand years, because it works. In our modern times the ideas you've studied here may not be widely discussed or accepted, but if you're honest with yourself, you have to admit they make a lot of sense.

It's not just that these ideas may apply to some small part of your life. They are pointing you to your entire destiny—to the very reason you came into this world—and now it's up to you to fulfill that destiny.

108 And So We Must See

IV.33–34 *The antidote of that moment
is the step where you finish off
the final end of the transformation.
Total purity is where those
who have grasped the emptiness
of the person and of things
develop each of the high qualities.
It too is something that comes
through the power of the mind,
for those who dwell in their own true nature.*

*Kshana pratiyogi parinama-aparanta
nigrahyah kramah.
Svarupa pratishtha va chiti shakter iti.*

We crave the idea of a beginning—it makes us feel more comfortable. Which came first, the chicken or the egg? Where did the first seed come from?

A seed is always planted by reacting to the product of an earlier seed: every person who has ever hurt you came from a seed that was planted when you hurt someone who hurt you before. There is no first seed, such a thing cannot be. We have been here forever, because we have always hurt back those who hurt us.

It seems like a cycle that could never be stopped. But one thing will save us: something we call a "spiritual antidote." If two ideas are struggling to win a single heart, and if one of them is false and the other is ultimately true, then truth will always prevail.

The ultimate antidote for all the pain of the entire world is emptiness: things that do things simply aren't there, and never were. We don't need to struggle with them anymore. We don't need to flail away at the bad man on the movie screen.

Things work only because they come from us, from our seeds—from taking care of each other.

Index of Important Ideas

(By Chapter and Verse)

Geshe Michael Roach is the first west-
erner in 600 years to pass the rigorous test for the title of Geshe, or Master of Buddhism, at Sera Mey
Tibetan Monastery, after twenty years of study in the
yoga and philosophy of India and Tibet. He is an hon-
ors graduate of Princeton University and has received
the Presidential Scholar medal at the White House.
Geshe Michael is the author of over thirty translations
of ancient texts, as well as books such as the international bestseller *The Diamond Cutter* and *The Tibetan Book
of Yoga*.

Christie McNally is a translator and
teacher of ancient Tibetan and Sanskrit texts. She is a
graduate of New York University, and has trained at
Tibetan monasteries in Nepal and India. She is a professor at Diamond Mountain University and has studied yoga extensively with some of the greatest Indian,
Tibetan, and western masters. She recently completed
the traditional Great Reatreat of three years, three
months, and three days in the high desert of Arizona.

The authors would like to express their special
thanks to Ms. Kimberley Veenhof, director of the Yoga
Studies Institute (YSI), for her constant encourage-
ment and assistance in completing *The Essential Yoga
Sutra*.

All proceeds from this book are being donated to
YSI, a nonprofit educational organization dedicated to
preserving the ancient manuscripts of yoga; translating
them; and presenting this authentic wisdom to the
modern world, in yoga schools and centers of all tra-
ditions, around the globe.

YSI provides seminars that bring alive the Yoga
Sutra—and other authentic ancient yoga classics and techniques. Please contact the Institute at *yogastudiesinstitute.
org* for information about having a YSI event at your
local yoga school or center.